QUIT SMOKING
&
NEVER
GO BACK

QUIT SMOKING
&
Never Go Back

PAUL ECCLES

Quit Smoking & Never Go Back:
A Guide to Quitting Smoking for Good

ISBN: 978-1-4716-7856-1

The author wishes to make clear that he is neither a qualified doctor nor any kind of healthcare professional. Therefore any advice given in this book is purely the opinion of the author and should not be used as a substitute for the medical advice of qualified persons. The reader should regularly consult their GP in regard to any symptoms that require treatment or diagnosis.

Front cover image: sippakorn / FreeDigitalPhotos.net

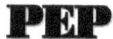

To my wife Laura and the kids.
Lots of love
xxxxx

Contents:

Introduction

'The believing we do something when we do nothing is the first illusion of tobacco.'

~Ralph Waldo Emerson

HELLO AND WELCOME – and congratulations. By reading this book you have taken the first of many positive strides towards quitting smoking and never going back. My name is Paul Eccles and I know very well what it is like to be addicted to smoking, to think you love cigarettes yet despise them. I spent more than fifteen long years stuck in the smoking rut and had started to believe I could never escape; that I was a prisoner for life. But I did escape. You can too.

The purpose of *Quit Smoking & Never Go Back* is to open your eyes to your smoking addiction – and yes, you are an addict, whether you like it or not. There are of course significant habitual elements to smoking, which we will look closely at later, but the root cause of smoking is your physical addiction. It is now time to see tobacco as it truly is. Whatever your preconceptions of smoking might be, leave them at the door. You need to look at cigarettes with a fresh pair of eyes – cast away the blinkers and look *really* hard. For as long as you have been a smoker you have been blinded by an ultimately simple yet highly effective piece of trickery. Through chemical addiction and psychological conditioning you are compelled to believe that smoking is not only rational but perfectly enjoyable. Believe me, it is neither.

I will share with you, through the course of this book,

how you too can quit smoking for good, without the endless pain and hardship so many of us seem to go through. If you've quit before and found yourself climbing the walls in frustration then you might find that statement hard to swallow. But don't worry. All will become clear as we continue.

However, to succeed in quitting smoking you need to bring along three things: an open mind, your undivided attention and a conviction that you no longer wish to smoke. That last requirement is especially important if you are to become a non-smoker. You have probably quit many times before and might be sceptical as to how I can help. That's understandable. And I'm going to be honest from the outset. Obviously, I am not magical in any way. Nor am I a miracle worker. Such people exist only in the realms of fiction and fantasy. I am a normal guy – a husband, a father, a son – who quit smoking and has had no inclination to go back. I smoked at least twenty a day (often a lot more) and thought I was trapped for life. But I found my way out. I solved the puzzle. With my advice, you can too.

I will not promise you anything nor make spurious guarantees. Don't get me wrong. It is my hope and belief that by reading this book you will escape nicotine addiction and never go back. I did it, and so can you. But it is down to you to implement what you learn. I will be there for you, but only as a positive voice in the background. Only you and you alone can quit smoking for yourself. I can't reach out from the book's text and pluck that cigarette from your lips (but I am working on it!). You are ultimately in control here. Together, though, I'm confident we will get you on the road to a smoke-free life.

I will not be asking you to rush out to the nearest

chemist and stock-up on nicotine patches and gum. Nor will I recommend pills or e-cigarettes or, for that matter, any other kind of smoking cessation product. You will be throwing away your cigarettes and breaking your smoking addiction through your own devices. I haven't got anything against these products, but I won't be asking you to use any of them.

I have written this book for all smokers, young and old. Whether you are in your sixties and smoking fifty-a-day or sixteen and smoking five, this book is for you. You are never too young or too old to quit. A smoker is a smoker. Of course, smoking is in many ways unique to each person – amount smoked per day, morning or evening smokers, choice of brand, etc. – but one thing binds all smokers together: nicotine addiction. Behind the engraved lighters and intricately patterned tobacco tins lies a chemical mechanism, and beyond that a psychological prison, that keeps all smokers lighting up.

I have endeavored to keep the chapters short and snappy and to avoid superfluous rambling – after all, perhaps you're waiting to start John Grisham's latest book. Don't worry; I won't keep you too long. Just long enough. The idea here is not to scoop a literary award but to get you to stop smoking tobacco for good. What you won't find in this book is endless exercises and 'grab a pen' moments. I will be honest now. I'm lazy and I don't like having to jump through hoops at a writer's behest. So I won't put you through that, either. I once started to read a 'quit smoking' book in which the author (who had never smoked) wanted to put me through weeks and months of exercises and games. I couldn't be bothered with that. All I need you to do is read on and let what I'm saying sink in. Similarly, this book isn't a set of military-style guidelines that must be scrupulously followed. Of course, you need to take heed of what I'm saying, but I have aimed for a relaxed, 'dip into' style. Once you have started reading, however, I would advise you not to drag it out for too long. Besides, provided you are deadly serious about quitting, you won't want to.

And there is one final point I should make. I am not going to take your cigarettes away from you. I am not going to suddenly make you throw them in the bin halfway through the book. Continue to smoke as you read, in whatever quantities you wish. In fact, continue to smoke after you read. There won't be any pressure from me. I will leave quitting up to you. I believe, though, that once you have read *Quit Smoking & Never Go Back* you will find yourself in an excellent position to quit happily.

Believe it or not, I have nothing against smokers. Each to their own. I'm not on a one-man mission to rid the world of tobacco addiction. My aim is to help those of you who desperately want to stop smoking yet find it tough to do so. If you want to smoke, then smoke. But, as with all things, perhaps it is better to do so knowing the truth.

It is my hope that, after reading, you will be on your way to a positive future as a non-smoker. This is one of the most important things you will ever do for yourself. This is about you. Quitting smoking is a priceless gift to bestow upon yourself. It's time to kick the cigarettes out for good and never go back.

So let's get going.

1. The World of Quitting Smoking

'The best way to stop smoking is to carry wet matches.'

~Anonymous

FOR MORE THAN FIFTEEN years of my life I smoked. That is to say that during those precious, irredeemable years I pumped my body full of toxic smoke to get from it the false sensations of pleasure and satisfaction. Quite how and why fate decreed that I should spend this period of my life chipping away at my health and fitness and well-being is a question I cannot answer. But that is the way it went. Some people escape it and some don't. If you are lucky enough to be one of those people who never started smoking, then never, ever go there. Any smoker will tell you why.

At first I enjoyed smoking, or, at least, enjoyed the relief smoking brought. Eventually, however, the realisation gradually dawned on me that I couldn't stop. Lighting a cigarette was a compulsion I could no longer control. It was a one-way street. What was worse, I could feel tobacco eating away at my confidence and looks and fitness. I began to see what all the fuss was about regarding quitting. I realized I had invited a monster into my midst. I first tried to quit when I was seventeen – an attempt that lasted mere hours before I buckled and headed to the nearest shop to secure a fix. That was my first crack at quitting smoking. There would be many more doomed attempts.

Over the years I have tried nicotine patches, gum, lozenges, pills, self-hypnosis, cold turkey and many more methods besides. Every attempt to quit seemed destined to end in abject failure. My biggest problem was that I couldn't imagine life without smoking. I was convinced that a life without smoking was a dull, boring life, a life of deprivation and joylessness. How wrong I was.

Quitting smoking is the biggest favour I ever did myself. After marrying my wife and fathering children, quitting is the greatest achievement of my life. I was in my early thirties when I stubbed out that final cigarette and I have never looked back. Up till then I was convinced – and utterly depressed because of it – that I was a confirmed smoker for life. I hated smoking, resented it for the seemingly inescapable prison it truly was to me back then. Every attempt I made to purge tobacco from my life resulted in the same miserable epilogue: a bruised return to smoking. There was nothing I could do about it, no weapon in my arsenal to defeat it. Nicotine had a hold over me so tight I felt suffocated, both physically and emotionally. I knew it would kill, or at least injure, me but still I persisted, helpless to escape.

But I did quit smoking. And I stayed a non-smoker. Nothing now could make me go back. I cannot tell you what a relief it is to be free from addiction, to be able to experience this one-off life without a portent of death and disease whispering in my ear. And it is my conviction that anyone can quit smoking and, more importantly, stay that way for life. Conventional wisdom says it is tough to quit. I disagree. It is we who make it difficult; it is we who throw up the barricades. But it doesn't have to be that way. With the right attitude and focus anyone – and I mean *anyone* – can say goodbye to cigarettes and never go back.

I consider myself to have been one of the very worst tobacco addicts. I was hopelessly hooked. In my time I have stooped unbelievably low to secure my next fix, shedding my scruples and sense of self-respect in the name of smoking – this supposedly enjoyable pastime. More than once I have fished stale dog-ends from an ashtray and rolled them into a foul-tasting emergency cigarette. I have even picked up damp dog-ends from my garden and tried to dry the tobacco in the microwave. I have stolen cigarettes from family and friends, often facing the ignominy of capture. I have lied and cheated in the name of tobacco. Yet still I persisted, bound as I was as an addict to secure my next fix.

I'm sure many of you, at some time, have too plunged the depths of indecency to be able to smoke. I'm sure most of you have at least been forced to cadge a cigarette from a stranger. I was sitting in a restaurant once with friends and, having no cigarettes and feeling itchy, asked a man on the next table if I could have one of his. He looked coolly at me for a moment, said simply, 'No,' and, with a sneer, returned to his conversation. Suffice to say I wanted the floor to swallow me whole. It's funny. I hear people say, 'I enjoy smoking.' I'm sure they enjoy eating, too. But I doubt you would find them rifling through a bin for a bit of stale pizza having been deprived of food for a couple of hours. And food, after all, is essential to life. Tobacco isn't anything of the kind, but we climb the walls when we can't have it, as though that next fag is as necessary as the very air we breathe. Where exactly does enjoyment come into it?

As I just said, food is essential to life and tobacco manifestly isn't. Right? Well, yes. But tobacco has some unusual properties. In later chapters I will show you how the addictive element of tobacco, nicotine, has got its feet under the table and made you regard it as indispensable. If you feel like I did when I was a smoker, then quitting must seem next to impossible – like trying to cross the Pacific in a dinghy. You may have quit before, perhaps holding out several weeks or even months. But each and every time, after much agonizing and soul-searching, you have gone back to cigarettes. I once quit for six months only to return miserably to smoking. The truth is that I never really left the addiction completely. Physically I might have been free, but the psychological dependency remained, strong and unyielding.

My attempts to quit smoking have varied considerably in duration. Like I said, six months was the longest I managed, time I spent largely fantasizing about lighting up and being an unmanageable grump. I've quit for a few months here, a few weeks there, too. Once, quite embarrassingly, I lasted twenty minutes. Honestly. I woke up and, like one does in a moment of clarity, declared myself a non-smoker. I started walking to work that morning and lit my 'last ever' cigarette, tossing the still half-full packet in a roadside bin. Twenty long minutes later I passed a shop and, after a few brief seconds of glum reckoning, stepped inside and bought some more. This is a classic example of an addicted mind at work.

This is what the serial quitter, as I was, goes through: this endless tug of war, this endless internal debate. You hate smoking, you really do. But as soon as cigarettes are removed from the equation smoking suddenly becomes more precious than air itself. Yet as you smoke that homecoming cigarette you ask yourself, 'Why am I doing this?' It is a cycle that will last a lifetime. I thought I couldn't break it. But I did. How? Well, that's what this book is about. I want to show you that you are not stuck with smoking. I want to show you that there is a way out. And most importantly, I want to show you that quitting smoking and never going back isn't the nightmare you probably think it is.

You have been programmed since birth to see smoking as many things: an essential social appendage; a stress reliever; a badge of sophistication; a perfectly normal thing to do. It isn't your fault you see smoking like this. We are the products of nature *and* nurture. We don't question everything; there just isn't time. Many things we simply have to accept. The trusty old cigarette is one of those things we never look at too closely. We know it is killing us yet we want it. Ridiculous? On the surface, yes. But peel back the layers and a subtle, devious and highly effective con trick will reveal itself.

The information in this book will, I hope, set you free. I won't make you any inflated promises. I won't claim that you *will* quit beyond any doubt. But I will say this. If you listen to what I'm saying, if you understand, then there is no reason whatsoever why you can't stop smoking. Don't be afraid. Just give it a go. Remember, I won't stop you smoking if you don't want to. But I suspect you'd love nothing more than to say goodbye to nicotine addiction once and for all.

If so, then welcome. You're in the right place.

2. Knowing Your Foe

'Smokers are like feet in ill-fitting shoes – they're always slipping out.'

~Anonymous

IF YOU'RE GOING to break free from smoking and never go back then it is essential you begin to look closely at why you smoke and, crucially, why you keep going back to it. To understand this you must first go back to the beginning.

Cigarettes are somewhat of a mystery to us. They were to me. They are produced by huge corporations that court little publicity yet turn over vast profits. The mystique of the cigarette, its aloof nature, is part of the reason you're hooked. You are forced to see it in a certain light. What do you really know about these finely chopped dried leaves encased in their paper tube? If you can understand every aspect of the cigarette – take a peek behind the stage curtain – you will soon be in a position to kick your addiction into touch.

Tobacco as we know it today comes from the leaves of *Nicotiana tabacum*, a perennial herbaceous plant native to Tropical America but now grown almost worldwide. It has been growing for several thousand years in the wild but now exists only in cultivation, in the vast tobacco plantations where the cigarette begins its journey. Tobacco shares the same family as the toxic *Atropa belladonna*, known more commonly as Deadly Nightshade. Crucially, the leaves of the tobacco plant contain, among other things, an alkaloid called nicotine, the chief chemical addictive element of the cigarette.

Tobacco use is nothing new. We can trace its roots back to the Native Americans, and before that the Mayans of Mexico. Tobacco, it seems, was more than simply a recreational drug. The leaves of the plant were used for medicinal purposes, acting as an antiseptic and painkiller. Tobacco also featured in shamanic rituals and was smoked through a pipe known as a calumet, or peace pipe. Clearly tobacco played a central role – spiritually and practically – in the traditions and ceremonies of Native Americans.

From the late 1400s onwards, European explorers began landing on the shores of the New World. One of those explorers was Christopher Columbus. He and his men would have been amongst the first Europeans to come into contact with tobacco. One of Columbus's crewmen, a Spaniard named Rodrigo de Jerez, is widely credited with being the first non-Native American tobacco smoker. Jerez even took some tobacco back to Spain where he was imprisoned by the pious Inquisition after being seen smoking, an alien concept at that time. Ironically, when he was released seven years later half of Spain was merrily puffing away.

Throughout the sixteenth century tobacco's popularity really gained a foothold. The great English seamen Sir Walter Raleigh and Sir Francis Drake were keen advocates of tobacco. Because of its addictive nature, tobacco's prominence grew rapidly, though for a while it remained the preserve of the wealthy. By the very late Elizabethan period this invidious plant was being cultivated in the New World by early tobacco barons and imported to Europe on a growing commercial basis, taking a firm and lasting grip within English society.

However, after the Virgin Queen died in 1603 she was succeeded by the James I, son of Mary, Queen of Scots, and for whatever reasons a staunch hater of tobacco. He even wrote a short book on his dislike called *A Counter-Blaste to Tobacco* in which he denounces the enterprise of tobacco smoking as 'base' and as a 'vile corruption'. There is, I suppose, even a vague reason to believe that King James's hate for tobacco ran so deep that his true motive for having Raleigh executed in 1618 was not due to his part in the treasonous Main Plot but instead that the latter was largely responsible for the introduction of smoking into polite society.

The modern cigarette, however, was not born until the late nineteenth century when a young inventor from Virginia named James Albert Bonsack, whose father was a plantation owner, invented the first cigarette rolling machine in answer to a competition. In 1881 Bonsack's revolutionary machine began to pump out cigarettes, not only in huge numbers but with incredible speed, effectively giving birth to the modern cigarette industry.

The rest, as they say, is history. From its obscure roots with the Native American tribes, tobacco usage now spread globally, wedging itself into popular culture, becoming part of every nation's psyche. Even during the great health scares of the Fifties and Sixties and the lawsuits of the Eighties, smoking continued to prevail. It is now estimated that there are in excess of a billion smokers worldwide. If you count in all those child smokers and occasional smokers, it could perhaps be closer to two billion. In other words, with 7 billion souls on our planet, around a quarter are addicted to smoking. I think that is just staggering.

But what is even more amazing is that it is a trick. It is smoke and mirrors on a grand scale. By combining the addictive nature of smoking with the tobacco giants' advertising and general media perception, the result is that a considerable chunk of humanity is convinced that smoking is enjoyable and indispensable. It is neither of those things. It is a life-threatening chemical addiction, a dependency that will last your entire shortened lifetime if you don't take positive steps to remove it.

The history of smoking could fill several thick volumes and of course I haven't the time to go into too much detail. But I hope you are starting to see that tobacco has no divine right to be in our lives. Humanity survived many thousands of years without needing a fag. Tobacco was an obscure plant growing in an obscure corner of the globe that was, through sailors and adventurers, introduced to our shores and the world beyond. From humble roots it has grown into a monster.

Knowing the cigarette intimately will begin to help you break your addiction to smoking. Once you know it inside out you will be able to see smoking for what it really is: a pointless chemical addiction and psychological dependency. Knowing where tobacco came from is one thing, but have you ever stopped and wondered what is actually *in* a cigarette? Given the health warnings, we might well suppose we know, more or less, what lurks inside that white paper casing. Yet seeing as we are inhaling tobacco smoke day in, day out, it is worth being totally clear on what we are digesting.

There is a little bit more to making the modern cigarette than rolling a bunch of raw leaves into paper, stuffing in a filter, and shipping them out to legions of waiting smokers.

There are many processes – drying, curing, fermentation – involved when it comes to producing the familiar modern cigarette, many of which rendering the tobacco more harmful and possibly even more addictive.

First of all, then, you must grow the tobacco plant. As mentioned earlier, you can find tobacco plantations in many countries the world over. Once the plant is harvested, the leaves go through a seemingly endless round of processing. Along the way additives are added to make the smoke from the cigarettes taste and smell more appealing, including sugar, menthol and various spices. One thing that isn't added is the nicotine, which occurs naturally in the plant. Nicotine is an organic compound, an alkaloid, and is a clear, thick, oily substance, highly poisonous, and the main addictive element of tobacco. In fact, I must point out that nicotine is a neurotoxin and its primary function within the tobacco plant is to poison anything that decides to try to eat it. The name nicotine comes from a sixteenth-century French ambassador to Portugal called Jean Nicot, who sent a package of tobacco seeds to Paris in 1550.

Yet the tobacco plant is home to more than just its *naturally* occurring poisons. From the soil the plant picks up many dangerous chemicals in the form of various insecticides and pesticides and fertilisers, which are sucked up and stored in the leaves. Arsenic – commonly used as rat poison – is one such chemical found in many fertilisers. DDT, a suspected carcinogen (cancer-causing), is often used as an insecticide. Trifluralin is a toxic chemical used in pesticides and is also believed to cause cancer. Every drag of a cigarette means you are ingesting these chemicals.

One particularly worrying entity attracted to the

tobacco plant is the metallic element polonium-210, which is highly radioactive. Dangerous amounts of it are collected by the tobacco plant, both from the soil and the air, and are breathed in when we smoke, delivering waves of damaging radiation to our lung cells. This idea that, as a smoker, I was breathing in radiation made me really think hard about my addiction and what I was doing to my precious body.

As if we needed them, even more carcinogens are added during the curing process, such as tobacco-specific nitrosamines, a group of strong cancer-triggering chemicals. And then, of course, there is the moment of lighting the cigarette. At this point, when the flame makes contact with the neat tip, an explosion of chemical reactions occurs. It is widely accepted that there are around 4000 chemicals in tobacco smoke, many of which spark into life upon the application of heat. Formaldehyde (which is used, among other things, to preserve dead bodies); Carbon Monoxide (which affects our ability to move oxygen around the body via our bloodstream); Tar (which is actually a sticky hotchpotch of particles responsible for all the staining and general clogging-up); Benzene (a well-known carcinogen, strongly linked with leukaemia); and ammonia (used as a toilet cleaner and apparently able to enhance nicotine's addictive powers).

Believe me, the list goes on. The cigarette is fit to burst with toxic chemicals – little wonder smokers are sadly far more likely to die from cancer. I hope you are beginning to see just what you have let yourself in for by becoming a smoker. That curling spiral of smoke hides an abundance of deadly sins. I'm not trying to scare you. But breaking away from smoking for good means facing up to the whole truth.

If you want to rid yourself of smoking then you are in the right place. I was lucky – very lucky – to see the truth about tobacco and quit for good. But there are innumerable smokers out there still trapped in the cycle of addiction. Don't be one of them for the rest of your life. I have written this book with the sole intention of helping you break away from cigarettes. It may not seem easy at the moment, but stick with me. By the time you have finished reading you will be in a unique position of power.

3. In the Beginning

'It has always been my rule never to smoke when asleep, and never to refrain when awake.'

~Mark Twain

WE SEE CIGARETTES from a young age. They are part of the fabric of the society that we grow up in. Smokers are everywhere. Of course, we have little concept when young of why adults are sucking back this smelly, eye-watering smoke from these strange white sticks, but nevertheless we accept it, as only a child can, as a fact of life. The way the world is.

In my case, my dad was a fairly heavy smoker. I grew up seeing him smoke and never really thought much about it (the only time I really paid attention to it was on the handful of occasions the hot tip accidently caught my arm or hand). I still have a vivid image of sitting in our lounge one idle Sunday afternoon, the television blaring in the background, watching him smoke a cigarette. The blue-grey smoke was curling up from the tip making these tortuously hypnotic patterns before dispersing into a vague mist near the ceiling. He genuinely didn't seem to notice he was smoking – he was just holding his smouldering papery stick as it burned inexorably towards his fingers.

Growing up in working-class, inner-city Birmingham, I was surrounded by tobacco use. There were many, non-immediate family members who smoked, not to mention friends and various other visitors to the house. Many of my friend's parents smoked, too. I was growing up in an environment where smoking was the done thing, the norm, a way of life. Ashtrays and lighters and dog-ends were a common and unquestioned sight. The smell of stale tobacco was nothing noteworthy. Little did I realise then that these experiences with cigarettes, these parading images, were conditioning me to smoke myself in later life – to fall prey to an addiction from which I would struggle to escape.

There comes a time when youngsters begin to question the adults about this strange activity called smoking. Even when it comes to something they have witnessed their entire lives, children's curiosity knows no bounds. They see adults doing it and ask:

Why are you smoking?
What are you getting from it?
Will I try it one day?

I recall hassling my dad about his smoking, only to be fobbed off with a half-baked mumble of uncertainty and a warning not to follow in his footsteps. My children questioned me about smoking, too, and I deflected their enquiries with the same aloofness exhibited by my dad. Because after all, what could I have said to them? I smoke because I'm addicted to nicotine, an alkaloid in the tobacco, which means I'm forced to take back this lethal mixture of chemicals to get my next fix? That would have made me sound like a fool …

Eventually, we reach an age where trying out cigarettes for ourselves becomes a possibility. I remember clearly my first dalliance with tobacco. I was a tender twelve years old when a friend of mine came to school on a cold morning brandishing a gold-coloured packet of cigarettes. I remember how they were arrayed in their neat ranks, partially hidden by a flap of paper. He offered me one there and then in the school playground and, perhaps egged on by the feral encouragement of assorted bystanders, I agreed.

We repaired to a quiet corner; he lit the cigarette and, after a few drags of his own, passed it over. I was more than a little apprehensive about this familiar, smoke-belching stick that I'd known all my life. I had known it only from a distance until now. But here I was, about to acquaint myself with the mysterious cigarette on a personal level. With a shrug and a nervous glance around, I took a drag and sucked back the smoke. Immediately I was plunged into a spluttering coughing fit as the fumes hit the back of my throat. I handed the vile thing back and vowed, amid a chorus of laughter, never to try that again. I honestly couldn't see the point.

Two years later, however, I accepted another cigarette – from the same friend (some friend, eh?) whilst sitting in a park one hot afternoon. Unsurprisingly, the initial result of the first drag was a bout of uncontrolled coughing. But I persisted this time. That afternoon, for reasons lost to me, I smoked three or four cigarettes, each one gradually less irritating. They didn't seem to do much for me – perhaps a vague boost, a slight kick.

Little did I realise what I had begun. From that point the seedlings of my affair with tobacco were sown in earnest. Before I left school I was, it seemed, irreversibly addicted, feeding the need for nicotine whenever I could lay my hands on a precious cigarette. Tobacco was, as it still is, expensive, so I resorted to slipping the occasional cigarette from my dad's packet. Otherwise, my pocket money was taken up almost immediately on the acquisition of cigarettes. When I look back, I cringe at the waste of money and at the breach of my parents' trust.

*

I started work at sixteen, joining a glazing firm in Birmingham. With a regular wage coming in I was now able to fund my addiction more thoroughly. I never saw it then as an addiction, of course, but as something, quite simply, one did; a pleasurable and widely indulged pastime. Eventually I started to drink in pubs. Everybody smoked: the bars of all drinking establishments were permanently semi-camouflaged by a screen of acrid tobacco smoke. This was before smoking was banned in 2007 in enclosed public places. Now smokers are forced to crowd outside to smoke. Have you ever seen someone standing outside a pub in the lashing rain, trying to smoke? Pleasure isn't a word that springs to mind.

Perhaps many of you will recall the first time you tried to quit smoking. At seventeen I had begun to realise that smoking had a downside – several downsides, in fact. Back then money was one of the driving forces of my attempts to quit smoking. My meagre wages were being eaten up too quickly by my need to purchase cigarettes. There was a very real sense that my hard-earned cash was quite literally disappearing in a puff of smoke. Already I was running short of funds before the week was out. This couldn't go on. I found myself borrowing money for cigarettes, a practice that continued for many years. Such is the ignominy of smoking.

My health, too, was a big concern. I was well aware of the horror stories of cancer and other killer illnesses, but at that age death seems like the preserve of the old. A more immediate concern was my worsening inability to play sports without tiring early. I used to play football quite regularly and keeping up the pace was becoming harder. After a few minutes I would be puffing away like an old horse. I knew it was the smoking. Even then, during what should have been my peak years, a tight chest, lack of breath and tickly cough were the norm. The cigarettes simply had to go.

But by then it was too late. I felt a strong sense of foreboding that ridding my life of tobacco wasn't going to be the walk in the park I'd imagined it would be. I began to resent cigarettes deeply. I wanted them. I needed them. But I hated them. A love-hate relationship was born, and would continue until I broke free for good.

4. The Truth About Smoking

'Cigarettes are killers that travel in packs.'

~Anonymous

WHEN I FINALLY quit smoking for good I was astonished by how simple it was. I'm not saying it was a complete breeze and that no effort was required, but compared with the common perception of the 'nightmare' of quitting smoking it was pretty easy. The battle I had expected never materialized. I made a binding vow that I would never smoke and stuck to it. I knew I couldn't carry on smoking. In my head had stubbornly lodged the idea that I wouldn't see my kids grow up, that I would be struck down by lung cancer or some other dreadful disease. Quitting was the only option.

The truth is that I only managed to quit smoking because of my many previous failures. Each time I buckled and went back to the cigarettes I learnt something new about myself and my addiction. Each failure was a lesson in quitting smoking for good – at least, that's how I now see it. Taking each of these experiences, I started to paint a detailed picture of smoking. The more I learned, the more real the possibility of success seemed. If you have quit many times before and always failed, don't worry. You will find those failures have taught you a lot.

So determined was I to see cigarettes off for good that the final time I quit I made it my business to understand in detail exactly why I smoked and why I couldn't give up.

This time, I vowed, quitting was for keeps, for life. I was sick of going back to the fags. The idea of never having to go back to smoking was taking root. I began to read about nicotine – what it is, how it works, and so on – and began to see the nasty chemical truth about smoking. The more I read, the more it seemed a door was opening, a door that would ultimately lead to freedom. But first I had to accept a harsh truth.

There is one bitter pill that must be swallowed if you are to break away from smoking, one point that you must unquestioningly accept. *You are a drug addict*. It is as simple as that. You probably already know this. But have you ever stopped and really thought about it. *A drug addict*. You are beholden to a substance, an external chemical that you must imbibe lest you begin to go half-mad. Accepting – and really *understanding* – that you are a drug addict is crucial to your success.

Drug addiction is a brain disease. Yes, a disease. Sufferers have the compulsive need for a given substance, in your case the nicotine contained within a cigarette. Often this need becomes uncontrollable. Even in spite of awful effects to their health, drug addicts will regardless continue to use. There is no cure. Once you have become addicted to a drug, relapse is always a possibility for the complacent. This you must accept here and now. You will always be a nicotine addict.

But don't worry. The good news is that this doesn't mean you need to continue to smoke. In fact, you never needed to smoke. With the right attitude, you will be able to face up to this addiction and move on. Armed with the truth about cigarettes, you will be able to leave smoking behind and never go back. All you need to do is read on with an open mind and a burning desire to be free.

*

Nicotine addiction is a con, a con you have fallen for. I con I fell for. A con that each of the world's one billion plus smokers are falling for every day. Nicotine, with its psychoactive properties, makes you believe whole-heartedly that smoking is a pleasurable experience and that you are receiving something essential to life. Furthermore, it creates feelings of itchiness and agitation if you don't keep your bloodstream topped up. Be clear on this: *you do not need to smoke. Full Stop.* You never needed it. You just think you do, thanks to the way nicotine works. The fact you were tricked, and remain tricked, is no reason to feel silly. Like I said, there are over a billion smokers in the world. You are far from alone.

As I was forced to smoke I often wondered how I had got into this mess. How had I ended up addicted to a drug? Smoking seemed so innocent in the early days. Well, we've seen how it starts, how society conditions us to see smoking through an obscure haze of mistruth. But think about it – really think! When we smoke, what do we do? We are setting fire to dried leaves and inhaling the fumes, ten, twenty, thirty times a day. Just let all the conditioning fall away a moment and really think about that. It is ridiculous, isn't it?

I started to think carefully about how I had been tricked into smoking. All around me, for as long as I remember, people had smoked. My brain was trained to accept it. But as I stood on the cusp of quitting for good I felt as if a grey cloud of deception was lifting away, revealing the truth. I could see smoking for what it was – a life-harming, malodorous, expensive waste of time. An addiction for life born of the chance chemical make-up of tobacco. Take away that all-important nicotine and what are you left with? The fumes from smoking dried leaves. That is all a cigarette is, but with a naturally occurring alkaloid within that keeps you hooked.

Once the penny drops, once you see smoking in its true light, you will be able to live your life without addiction. What causes all the 'pain', what causes the 'distress' when quitting smoking is holding on to those false beliefs, those preconditioned ideas. You have put smoking on a pedestal, made it precious. Once you can look tobacco in the eye and understand it, you will let it go. It may not feel that way at the moment. But read on. It soon will.

5. Why can't I stop smoking?

'Smokers don't get to smoke. They have to smoke.'

~Anonymous

COME RAIN OR SHINE, be they good times or bad, you have to smoke, whether you want to or not. You have probably attempted to stop before but eventually, after much miserable inner debate, crawled back to tobacco once again. Like I said, the only way to quit smoking and never go back is to understand why you smoke, to really get to the heart of your addiction. There are two main elements to your smoking addiction and it is only by fully appreciating both of them that you will be able to quit for good.

The first is the physical side of your addiction. Remember, you are addicted to nicotine, the naturally occurring alkaloid in tobacco and one of the most addictive substances known to humanity. You are just one of over a billion smokers globally, all of whom are compelled to use tobacco, to poison themselves, over and again. Nicotine makes you feel as though you are receiving something pleasurable. Of course, you manifestly are not. You are in fact self-administering a lethal cocktail of chemicals that is gunging up your body and in all likelihood bringing forward your death by years. Your humble coffee-time companion is, in truth, a ruthless killer. The cigarette is simply nicotine's delivery system, a system that requires you to breathe in poisons to receive the drug. Sorry to be so blunt, but if you want to escape then you need the facts. The truth, as they say, will set you free.

You are trapped in a cycle of chemical dependency. When you don't smoke you become itchy and restless and agitated. The cigarette briefly relieves these feelings and seems to return you to a state of calm. Does that mean all those non-smokers out there are suffering these same uncomfortable sensations and could easily get rid of them by smoking? Of course not. Only smokers suffer like this. The only way to crush this itchy desire for a cigarette is to stop smoking, but the nature of nicotine is making that very difficult for you presently. Don't worry. With the right knowledge you can set yourself free.

The other side of our addiction is perhaps the more difficult to understand; it is the behavioural side of smoking, the emotional side, the habitual side. Since taking that first drag of that first cigarette you have being spinning a complex web of associations, i.e. moments and occasions when you get an urge to light up. Combined with the false chemical 'high' we receive when smoking, our experiences in life have given us a series of smoking triggers, moments when the notion of smoking seems even more precious than normal. Common ones are the first cigarette of the day, or the one with tea or coffee, or the one after a long car trip. But the list is almost endless, and each one of us has built up our own unique pattern of smoking behaviour.

It is this emotional dependence on smoking that is the harder part of your addiction to break. If we refrain from smoking, nicotine is virtually gone from our body within a few days, meaning the psychical side of the cravings has already vanished. But the associations we have constructed over time mean we crave cigarettes for a long time after quitting. Some people I've spoken to have been craving cigarettes years after quitting. But don't worry. With the right attitude I'm sure you won't be one of them.

If you are going to break free from cigarettes once and for all, it is imperative you understand your addiction inside out. If you want to defeat an enemy, knowing the way it works is essential, and quitting smoking is no different. Since the first time you smoked, the physical addiction to nicotine and the psychological dependency have been working in harmony to keep you hooked. They are the perpetrators of a clever trick that has you fooled. But not for much longer.

First, let's look at the physical side of the addiction.

6. The Mechanics of Tobacco Addiction

'Cigarettes are like an old friend, but one that wants you dead.'

~Anonymous

I'M SORRY BUT YOU'VE been duped. Conned. Led a merry dance. Tobacco isn't what you think it is. The faithful cigarette is not what you think it is. Is it pleasurable to smoke? No, it isn't. It may seem that way, but it is not. To understand how the wool has been pulled over your eyes, you need to understand how nicotine invades your brain and creates the illusion of pleasure and satisfaction.

At the very centre of the smoking world is nicotine addiction. Forget fancy engraved lighters. Forget novelty ashtrays and Audrey Hepburn-style cigarette holders. And forget flavoured cigarette papers. All these appendages serve as nothing more than the respectable face of your life-threatening addiction to tobacco and, more specifically, nicotine.

So what actually happens when we smoke? How does nicotine keep us coming back for more? It is a simple yet subtle trick, a chemical illusion. But do not doubt its power. Remember, there are perhaps as many as two billion smokers in the world, each one of them falling for tobacco's bitter lies time and time again. To understand things clearly, we need to look at exactly what happens as we breathe in that blast of smoke.

As soon as we take that first drag of a cigarette and suck it back most of the tobacco smoke rushes straight to our lungs. There the nicotine is absorbed into our bloodstream by the alveoli, tiny air sacs that resemble a bunch of grapes and are responsible for gas exchanges. From there nicotine hitches a ride in our bloodstream to our brain. On its way it passes the blood-brain barrier, a kind of checkpoint at the entrance of the brain that prevents anything undesirable from entering. However, as with other psychoactive drugs, nicotine molecules are small enough to get through and proceed unhindered.

Now those nicotine molecules are in our brain. About seven seconds have elapsed since that first drag. Now nicotine can get to work. Our brains are full of neurotransmitters, chemical messengers that whizz around passing messages between neurons. Neurotransmitters fit into receptors on the surface of nerve cells, like a key going into a lock, and thus regulate bodily functions.

There is one neurotransmitter in particular called acetylcholine that regulates various processes, such as memory and breathing and muscle movement. Acetylcholine is essential to the way nicotine operates. Like I've said throughout this book so far, smoking is a trick, and the first part of the trick happens here at the chemical level. Nicotine, you see, is an imposter, a master of disguise. Nicotine's chemical make-up is, purely by coincidence, uncannily similar to that of acetylcholine. Given this likeness, nicotine molecules are able to dock comfortably into those receptors usually occupied by acetylcholine. It is like a burglar with a key to your house.

Once safely ensconced in these receptors, nicotine mimics acetylcholine, but not very well – after all, it's not the real thing. We also see an increase in the amount of receptors as the brain tries to cope with the abundance of what it thinks is acetylcholine, a process called upregulation. The nicotine's presence starts releasing other neurotransmitters, but with gleeful abandon. This is how nicotine creates its effects. The neurotransmitters released have a psychoactive affect on our minds. Epinephrine, known commonly as adrenaline, is let out of the traps, giving us a sense of alertness, of 'flight or fight'. Beta endorphin is released, too. This is a natural opiate and can bring about a sense of calm and relaxation.

One crucial neurotransmitter released in high quantities is dopamine, and it is nicotine's misuse of dopamine that lies at the heart of the trick. Dopamine, you see, is responsible for our body's reward system. When you sate your appetite with food, the good feeling you receive is the work of dopamine. When you receive good news, that feeling of elation is dopamine. When you're bursting for the toilet and finally manage to relieve yourself, that sense of satisfaction is, you might have guessed by now, dopamine.

Dopamine's function is to reward positive behaviour, behaviour beneficial to our existence. We need to eat, right? Well dopamine helps make eating pleasurable to reinforce the activity. Without that feeling of pleasure eating would fall down our list of priorities, which wouldn't be good for our well-being. During sex we receive a blast of dopamine, ensuring at a primal level the continuation of the species. Our bodies need rest, too, so dopamine is released when we find time to relax.

But if nicotine is causing a release of dopamine then that means we are in essence being rewarded for smoking. Do you see? Yet smoking is not a pleasurable experience. Cigarette smoke is packed with poisonous gases and carcinogens and irritating gases. Even with all the additives the tobacco companies pack into cigarettes they are still vile. Ever got smoke in your eye? Not nice, is it? Or have you ever choked on tobacco smoke? Again, there is nothing remotely nice about that. Cigarette smoke is foul. But that doesn't matter. The dopamine is telling us it is good. It seems to smokers that smoke from a cigarette is beneficial and desirable.

Our reward pathways have been taken over by nicotine. We are getting a sense of pleasure from something totally unpleasant. Think about it. A cigarette never seems more revolting than during a cold or flu. Yet why is it we puff our way through such illnesses, even though doing so is horrendous, even painful? Each drag is a burden on our raw throat yet on we go. Why? Because our brain is telling us that doing so is pleasurable and beneficial to our existence. We consciously know it isn't, but if we can't rely on our instincts …

Nicotine has something called an elimination half-life, in other words the amount of time taken for the drug to be reduced by half in the bloodstream. This half-life is about an hour or so. As nicotine is metabolized by the liver we begin to feel that familiar itch. *I need a cigarette* is how we interpret it. Common withdrawal symptoms from nicotine are restlessness, agitation, depression, poor concentration; the list goes on. But we know these symptoms well, because we feel them whenever we want a cigarette.

If you are made to wait to smoke, you become restless. Whenever I used to go for a meal with my wife and kids I would begin to get fidgety because I couldn't smoke. Eventually I would have to disappear outside to have a crafty fag. These feelings of irritation are caused by nicotine's reduced presence in our bloodstream. Therefore we introduce a fresh batch of nicotine to repel them. This cycle goes on and on and on.

I said earlier that non-smokers don't feel this mental torture – they haven't got to endure this itchiness brought about by nicotine. But as a smoker, you are driven to light up throughout the day, again and again, to stave off these creeping feelings of unease. You light a cigarette and get your fix of dopamine and the restlessness subsides. But not for long.

Up till now you have probably seen smoking as a trusty friend, something to lean on when times get tough. But it isn't any such thing. *The cigarette has caused you to feel like this. The bad mood and fidgeting are down to smoking. Stop smoking and they will go away in time.*

Sucking back the fumes of dried tobacco leaves is not going to improve your life. How could it? From now on you must start seeing tobacco as it is: dried leaves encased in paper that you set fire to and whose fumes you inhale. Those dried leaves contain a sticky alkaloid that causes you to become an addict, for life. Doesn't sound too good, does it?

With the right attitude and knowledge quitting smoking can be fairly straightforward. At the moment you probably still see smoking as a positive behaviour. But are you starting to see? It's just illusory, a con trick. The alkaloid nicotine is fooling you into believing you're getting a reward. You need to have the true picture of smoking planted firmly in your mind. Once you can see it clearly you will be one step closer to a life without addiction

Although the actual physical mechanism of nicotine addiction pulls us down, what really keeps us there is the other side of our addiction. The psychological side of smoking is a tangled jungle of associations and triggers and illusions that together make a seemingly impenetrable barrier. But as you will see, it doesn't have to be so.

7. Psychological Warfare

'I don't mind being a statistic – just not a dead one.'

~Anonymous

WERE SMOKING A simple case of physical addiction, I truly believe that there would be hardly any smokers left in the world. If every smoker utterly disliked smoking and fully understood the addiction, smoking simply to answer the physical yearning, there would be no need for this book. But there most certainly is a need. There is a need because smoking soars far beyond a straightforward chemical addiction.

The psychological dependence on smoking, to which every smoker is prey, is the real driving force behind our inability to quit smoking. That is not to say that physical addiction to nicotine doesn't play a role. It is this initial addiction to the feeling nicotine offers us that sees us become addicts. In a sense, the physical addiction leads us into the deception. Once we are hooked, however, the reins are passed over. Nicotine addiction gives birth to a beast: a psychological dependence on smoking. Our physical addiction now takes a backseat and lets our warped minds perpetuate the falsehood.

If we really take the time to analyze the physical addiction, there isn't that much to it. We imbibe nicotine and receive a brief boost, a fleeting return to calmer waters. But after a while, the nicotine in our system decreases, leaving us feeling itchy and fidgety. So we smoke another cigarette to receive another boost and remove the discomfort once again. Simple.

But allow me to make a point here. Let us imagine that drinking battery acid offered the same mechanism, the same mode of entrapment. Let us imagine there were certain people out there drinking battery acid to get a fix. Would you try it? Of course not. The mere notion is unimaginable. Just think how disgusting, how poisonous it would taste, how it would burn your throat. Now imagine that you knew fully well that drinking the battery acid tricks you into believing it is satisfactory and pleasurable, and that it causes agitation and itchiness that can be curtailed only by ingesting more battery acid, hence creating a toxic, lifelong cycle. Can you imagine falling into this trap? Never. You would want to shake these addicts by the lapels and compel them to stop – tell them they don't have to do it.

But don't you see? You are in a similar position with smoking, only cigarettes are socially acceptable – even non-smokers' minds are warped by society's perception of smoking. No one could easily be fooled into drinking battery acid. But then battery acid hasn't been the subject of advertising campaigns promoting its plus points. We don't see Hollywood stars onscreen drinking it. Our minds aren't programmed to believe what we hear about it.

Now don't get me wrong. Of course battery acid has no properties that can addict you to it, physical or psychological. But the point here is that cigarettes *do* have a psychoactive effect, which has combined with the endless conditioning you've received since birth to ensure you see a cigarette as completely normal. In fact, if battery acid worked like nicotine does and was thrust upon us by the media and advertisers, a few desperate souls actually would be taking it. (In fact, I'm sorry to say this, but tobacco smoke contains cadmium, which happens to be a component of battery acid.)

Take methamphetamine (crystal meth), for instance, a highly addictive psychoactive drug whose effects on long-term users can be quite horrific. Who in their right mind would want to become a meth addict? Would you want to be beholden to crystal meth, forced to smoke it or, worse, inject it? Common side effects of meth use include acute weight loss, psychosis, 'meth mouth' (in which your teeth fall out) and in harsher cases brain damage and death. Most of us would be utterly appalled and terrified by the thought of taking methamphetamine, but that is because, like battery acid, we haven't had a wealth of propaganda thrown at us for years, espousing its advantages. After all, is a cigarette all that much better? Not really. Smoking can cause your teeth to fall out by way of gum disease. And death is always a concern for smokers: lung cancer, heart disease, chronic obstructive pulmonary disease … Remember, a cigarette is nothing more than the leaves from a tobacco plant, cured, chopped, dried and rolled inside a paper tube. You set fire to the leaves, suck back the smoke and your brain is assaulted by nicotine, the neurotoxin in the tobacco plant's leaves that it uses to prevent insects eating it. That's it. Nothing more.

If you are to quit smoking and never go back it is essential you start seeing the cigarette in this true light. Let everything you believed until now wash away to reveal the truth. You just need a little focus. Practice this whenever possible: every time you pluck a cigarette from its box look at it carefully. Forget the fancy packaging. Look solely at that fag and think about what it is – *all* it is. Next time you see a smoker, see them for what they are: an addict who has been tricked. Smell the smoke and ask yourself whether you really want to spend the rest of your life breathing it into your precious lungs.

This new way of thinking will set you free. Trying to see something in a new light isn't always easy, which is why you must start now. By the time you quit it will be second nature. Have you ever read a novel in which there is a huge twist in the final chapter? The twist changes everything. Every character, every scene is now cast in a new light. If and when you read that book again, will you be fooled? No. You will interpret what you read in light of the truth you know is revealed at the end. You won't fall for the red herrings a second time.

Smoking is no different. You are a product of the society you have grown up in. That society has wrongly told you smoking is pleasurable and rewarding when it isn't. The way nicotine works has reinforced the fraud. But now you know it is a mistruth, a cunning deception. Don't continue to fall for it. Move away from the smoke and the staining and the coughing into the fresh air and see the simple truth.

All smokers have those times of day when a cigarette seems extra precious. My 'favourite' cigarette was always the one with a cup of tea. But why did that cigarette seem more valuable than the others I smoked throughout the day? It all comes back to the psychological conditioning. We are, of course, physically addicted to nicotine, but it is our warped view of smoking, our addicted minds, which make quitting so tough – when it doesn't have to be.

I now know I had no choice but to smoke those cigarettes with my tea. I was craving the nicotine. My brain was crying out for its reward, for its shot of dopamine and an end to the restlessness of nicotine withdrawal. When I look back it is so clear, so simple. But at the time I genuinely thought I enjoyed that smoking break. In fact, I did. But not the smoking part. The break itself was a genuine pleasure; a break from work, a chance to rest.

But because I had been busy I had naturally abstained from smoking, which meant the restlessness and yearning for a cigarette were reaching fever pitch. Non-smokers enjoy a break just as much. They put the kettle on and sit down. Smokers do the same, but before they can relax they have to get a fix of nicotine to reduce the agitation brought about by their addiction. Do you see how a cigarette has tainted that rest break and not improved it? The cigarette was just a necessity. It didn't enhance the break – it just made it bearable.

Another interesting aspect of the tea- and coffee-based associations is that these drinks are very effective at rendering the cigarette more tolerable. I would in fact go as far to say that smoking and hot beverages go hand-in-hand for this reason above all others. Just think about it. Have you noticed that smokers always seem to have a mug in their hands? The kettle is always on. A fresh round of coffee is always imminent. This is because smoking cigarette after cigarette is not a pleasant thing to do. Even with all the additives, smoking one cigarette after another is awful. By pairing smoking and drinking, the hot liquid in part reduces the smoky rawness in our throat left by the cigarette.

Remember, we don't smoke for the taste. No one does. If smoking wasn't highly addictive there would not be a smoker left in the world. Smokers smoke to get the drug within, driven on by a warped mind. That is it. Any other reason is nothing more than a flimsy rationalization.

But what about all those other times during the day that we smoke? In the morning, in the car, after housework. I even used to smoke in the bath! We smoke because we are addicted to nicotine and psychologically dependent on tobacco. No other reasons. Our addicted brains require that dose of dopamine to make us feel better, to give us a reward. We don't *need* it – in fact smoking is destroying our health – but that is the nature and the wrath of the trick we have unwittingly fallen for. This constant need to replenish our nicotine levels has endowed us with a mesh of behaviours, of associations and triggers. We have come to recognise certain times as being inextricably linked with tobacco.

Like I said, my time, among others, was a cup of tea. As soon as that kettle went on, I craved nicotine; I had come to expect my reward during this time. In fact, the first cup of tea of my day is always a pleasurable experience anyway, with or without nicotine. But as a smoker I couldn't enjoy that moment without bolstering it with a dose of dopamine, on top of that I got naturally, and putting an end to the agitation. Do you see?

Have you noticed that the really popular triggers are always forged through abstinence? The cigarette in the morning? You just need a fix after going a full ten hours or so without nicotine. After a long car journey? Getting that fix after hours of deprivation. After a meal? After work? These are simple Pavlovian principles at play. Like Pavlov's hungry dogs salivated at the clanging of a bell, our subconscious minds begin to get hungry for nicotine right on cue. If you are going to quit smoking and never go back, then you will need to break these associations, sever the link that keeps you lighting up

Social occasions are a big test for quitters, especially those times involving alcohol. You will doubtless have built up a network of considerably strong associations at these times. Not only will every regular smoker be puffing away like a chimney stack, but those who don't usually go near a cigarette will be smoking too. These situations in which you are surrounded by alcohol and blasts of smoke are often enough to push you over the edge. How many times have you buckled and smoked during such events? I know I have, many times.

But again, it is very much about perspective. Just think about those people puffing away with abandon. In the morning they will wake up with raw throats and tight chests. Their clothes and hair and skin will be saturated with cigarette smoke. They will, in that moment, wish they were a non-smoker like you – especially as they reach automatically for their fags, rueing the fact they must smoke them.

See all those smokers as they really are: addicts. Ignore all your previous preconceptions about smoking. Enjoy your evening without having to light up every ten minutes. Enjoy your evening without worrying whether you will have enough cigarettes to see you through. Enjoy your evening without having to meekly ask a stranger if you can have one of their cigarettes. Enjoy your evening without being conscious of how you reek of stale smoke. Enjoy your evening without that nagging voice telling you it is yet again time to inhale smoke to get a fix. Will you really miss smoking at these times? I certainly don't.

Smoking sinks into the very fabric of our existence. It is ingrained in our shared psyche. We buy gold-plated petrol lighters and customised tobacco tins. We have novelty ashtrays and flavoured cigarette papers. Smoking becomes one of the defining characteristics of our lives. But it isn't our fault. We have been led to believe the lies about tobacco through the warped image of smoking we are offered by society at large.

And nowhere is the image of smoking more played upon than in film and television. Since the very birth of motion pictures, the cigarette has been used as a prop to seemingly enhance the characters on-screen. When I was growing up I loved the *Die Hard* films with Bruce Willis. Still do, as it happens. His character John McClane is always pitted against such difficult odds, his chances so overwhelmingly slim, yet always he comes through and saves the day in his own wisecracking way. Whenever there is a lull in the bad-guy killing, he snatches a cigarette and lights it with a Zippo-style lighter. This image was one that sunk deep into my soul: this hard-bitten cop, fighting impossible odds, taking a well-deserved cigarette break. When I was around fifteen I bought a similar lighter and, embarrassing as it is, even remember smoking with the same mannerisms as my hero.

What I didn't know, of course, was that the character in the film was trapped in the same cycle I was. He wasn't smoking because he wanted to but because he *had* to. Not only did he have to battle a crew of psychopathic international terrorists, but he was doing so with the agitating effects of nicotine withdrawal. He craved that reward, that release of dopamine, like all smokers. It was nothing more than drug addiction dolled up to appear macho and glamorous. I fell totally for that image. Yet perhaps the smoking made the film. After all, without all those smoking breaks he might have picked off the bad guys far too quickly for the director's liking!

And it is not just to add machismo that cigarettes are employed by filmmakers. Take Audrey Hepburn in *Breakfast at Tiffany's*. Remember the velvet gloves and, more importantly, the long slender cigarette holder? That is now an iconic movie image, an encapsulation of femininity and sophistication. But think about it. She is being forced to inhale chemical-laden smoke through addiction. Would she smell of perfume or stale smoke? Would she still exude the same glamour after her teeth have fallen out through gum disease? There is nothing feminine or sophisticated about smoking, however much the movie people try to say there is.

It is not just to enhance stereotypical features of the sexes that smoking is employed. Have you ever seen one of those war movies where the dying soldier has a cigarette thrust in his mouth by one of his well-meaning comrades? There is in fact evidence that smoking can reduce pain, by way of the beta-endorphin that is released. But so can painkillers, far more effectively. Any pain relief from smoking is transient and slight and certainly not capable of washing away the agony of a mortal wound. Yet that dying soldier sucks on that cigarette like it is a slice of pure joy. The soldier is simply an addict like any smoker, but you can see how powerful an image like that is and how it sticks.

There is a glut of television programmes in which the characters spend every moment smoking away. For years on Britain's two most popular soap operas, *Coronation Street* and *Eastenders*, many of the characters smoked almost non-stop. To be fair, though, in recent times this has been reduced considerably. Yet the cigarette still remains the ultimate TV prop. If characters are stressed, give them a cigarette. If a puzzle needs solving, send in the cigarettes. In Pain? Have a fag. Relaxation? You guessed it. We are bombarded with this imagery every day. Moreover, our children are, too, producing the next generation of warped minds, of lambs to the slaughter.

Every cigarette smoked by every film or television character has been done so for dramatic effect, based on the incorrect understanding that smoking is beneficial and helpful. It is neither. It is a drug addiction with strong habitual elements. It is harmful to one's health and totally unnecessary. Don't keep falling for the trick.

8. *The Reality of Cravings*

'I'll smoke anything anybody gives me, I'm not particular.'

~Peter Falk

CRAVINGS. THOSE TEAR-YOUR-HAIR-OUT moments that see many well-intentioned quitters return bruised and battered to smoking. It always comes back to cravings. It is the mechanism of cravings that keep you lighting up. They can strike seemingly from nowhere, crippling your mind and ripping away the fortifications you have built to prevent relapse. Whenever we encounter someone in the process of quitting smoking, they will often remark on how bad the cravings are. It is the acute fear of these so-called cravings that keep smokers lighting up.

So how, in that case, are you going to quit smoking if you are being perpetually bombarded with mind-bending urges to smoke? Like with most principles in this book, it is a question of perception. Cravings don't have to be a nightmare. In fact, they can even be useful. But the only way to come to terms with cravings is to understand them and to strip away some of the myths surrounding these moments of apparent agony.

So, what is a craving? The best way to explain it is as a powerful desire for something, in this case a cigarette. The feeling is best described as a kind of emptiness, a knot of anxiety joined with a powerful feeling of *I want a cigarette*. When a craving hits we get an often uncontrollable urge to light a cigarette. As a smoker, you

44

should know this feeling well. Cravings are not the preserve of those trying to quit. You experience cravings all the time. Every time you are placed in a position in which you cannot smoke, at some point that familiar tug of anxiety will prevail. Whenever you reach for a cigarette it is the result of a craving, however slight. Cravings are nothing new to you and certainly nothing to be scared of. You get them all the time, only presently you are lighting up and feeding fresh nicotine into your system to keep the beast at bay. Your cravings are nothing to be bothered about because you can staunch them.

But once you quit you cannot quell these moments by reaching for your cigarettes. That is no longer an option. Well, it is an option, but one you have no wish to take. So you hold out and try to be brave. These urges get stronger and more intense and you begin to realize you have a real battle on your hands. Unless you are possessed of unworldly strength of character, at some point the urge is just too strong and you smoke. You regret it, of course, but there wasn't another way to beat off the agitation. Funny, isn't it, how when we quit smoking we see lighting up as simply not an option and finish by seeing it as the *only* option?

There is no single, irrefutable scientific answer to what a craving is. In truth, a 'craving' is just the term we lend to the want for nicotine, the need or desire for a cigarette. The ailing presence of nicotine in your body will of course trigger a craving. This is the mechanism that keeps you trapped. But what about those cravings that are experienced weeks and months after quitting? Given that your body is effectively free from nicotine within a few days, these cravings cannot possibly be attributed to falling nicotine levels. They can only be psychological.

The root of our cravings lies in our perception of smoking. I have spent countless hours pondering this and have arrived at the conclusion that a craving is brought on by our own romantic view of cigarettes. If you have tried to quit before and failed then you might understand. I was often weeks into quitting and would quite suddenly be besieged by an agonizing urge to light up. But crucially this urge was preceded by thinking about smoking. For instance, I would walk past a pub and see a group of smokers puffing away outside. Immediately I would begin to fantasize about being among their number, how nice it would be to join them. Forget the raw throats and smelly clothes and chesty coughs. The idea of smoking would become suddenly very precious, and as a result I felt a wave of anxiety that I could not partake.

Do you see what I am saying? There is no outside influence causing our cravings. There is no physical entity acting as a puppet master to our urges. The root cause isn't physical but psychological. That initial psychological trigger causes a range of symptoms such shaking, sweating, anxiety, depression and nausea. Our emotional dependence on smoking is so strong that we are forced to bear these moments of trauma, these *cravings*.

When I quit for good, I still experienced cravings, but they didn't bother me. Every time a stray thought of smoking triggered an urge to smoke, my rational mind would squash it. I could see exactly what smoking was and how I had been duped by it. I wasn't fooled anymore. Cravings became almost a good thing. They were a sign that I was slowly healing my mind.

I was clinical in my approach to cravings. When one hit me, I immediately analyzed the feeling. After doing this for a while I came to realize there was nothing to them.

The actual physical sensation of a nicotine craving is nothing to worry about: slight tension; an empty feeling; a vague lightheadedness. I knew these sensations were what I had to bear for a while if I wanted to be free from tobacco. Besides which, as a smoker I regularly went through these moments when unable to smoke. Remember, the real 'agony' of cravings is all in the mind. *You* are the sole manufacturer of your urges to smoke. *You* ultimately put smoking on a pedestal.

By changing your mind-set, any cravings you receive will hardly bother you at all. Don't worry about the physical symptoms; they are nothing. Your perception of smoking – the correct perception – is the key to beating cravings. See these moments for what they are and they will pass. Use cravings as a positive. This is the healing process; your mind is coming round to its new reality. But it will take a little time to adjust.

When a craving struck, I was prepared for it. You too need to be prepared. As much as you can see cigarettes in their true colours, at some point you will think about smoking. This will trigger a craving. What you do next is critical. First, take three or so deep breaths. Make them really deep abdominal breaths, taking in the air slowly through your nose until your lungs are full and then slowly exhaling. This will help create a sense of calm. Deep breathing releases endorphins – a kind of natural opiate – and will create a sense of well-being. Try it now. It works.

Once you have taken these breaths, take a moment to think about smoking as a whole. Think about everything you now know about cigarettes: where they come from, how they work, how you have been conned by them. This will help create a sense of perspective. After you have done this, think about the craving you are experiencing.

Ask yourself whether it is really *that* unbearable. You will find it isn't and that you can easily deal with it.

Finally, think about how much you desire a life without tobacco. Think about that quarter of the world's population trapped. Do you want to be one of them for the rest of your days? Of course not. You finally want to beat this terrible addiction and once again become the master of your own destiny.

As time goes on you will develop automatic responses to cravings. You will be armed with the truth and cigarettes will be powerless to tempt you back into the fold. The average craving, so conventional wisdom has it, lasts 3-5 minutes. This is about right. But I know through experience it can seem much longer than that if you are in the wrong mind-set. Yet with the right approach cravings will quickly become less frequent and less intense and will disappear almost completely.

Having said that, even now I get the occasional craving. Remember that a craving is created by a thought of smoking, a stray reminiscence. We are all addicts, don't forget. Even though those receptors have reduced in number, there are still traces of our addiction remaining in the depths of our subconscious. They will never go. When I get the very occasional – and I mean *very* occasional – craving, it actually makes me smile. It reminds me of where I was back then and where I am now. I don't worry about it. My mind is long-hardened to not smoking. Who knows? In time maybe these random urges will disappear forever.

As long as you keep in mind that cravings are harmless, temporary and a natural part of the road to freedom, they really will not bother you. The idea of cravings being highly traumatic is perpetuated by society.

It is an accepted fact, even though it is not quite true. *It is all about perception*. You are now in a position of power. You are starting to see smoking with the blinkers removed. Whatever you do, never go back to those days of ignoreance.

9. Flirting with Danger

'Health is not everything, but without health, everything else is nothing.'

~Anonymous

WE ALL KNOW THE dangers of smoking, don't we? Every cigarette packet carries a bold warning regarding the dangers of sustained tobacco consumption. We all know someone or have heard of someone who died of a smoking-related disease. But what are the real risks? Are they overstated? Or is smoking tobacco really the death sentence it is portrayed to be?

Perhaps the greatest thing about quitting smoking is the peace of mind it brings in terms of our health. Our health is without question the most important asset we own. There are doubtless many sick millionaires who will testify as such. Even those smokers who have no intention of quitting and are, they insist, perfectly happy, will concede that the damage the smoke is doing to their health is a cross they are reluctant to bear.

But health never comes in to it when you are an addict. If cigarettes were not addictive there would be very few, if any, smokers left in the world. We smoke because we have to, because we are addicts. It is that simple. And addicts will continue to use in the face of terrible consequences to their health. Think about it. We are rational people. Smoking apart, what other activity do we partake in that has a good chance of killing us, or at least shortening our life? None, if we can help it. You don't want to die; I don't want to die. We want to live, to experience this unique chance to exist and to understand our world, to watch our children grow up.

But smoking flies in the face of this desire, doesn't it? We know fully well smoking might kill us. We know for certain that it will clog up our bodies and rob us of health and fitness – that much has already begun. But still we persist, puffing away, piling excuse upon excuse as to why quitting isn't an option in the near future. I recall only too clearly wanting to give up smoking yet never feeling the time was right. Without the right attitude, the time will never be right. Ever.

I hope you can sense, in the recesses of your mind, a glimmer of a chance forming, a chance to walk away from the addiction you hate yet cannot live without. If you can't, don't worry; there is time aplenty.

I was in two minds about going into great detail about the effects tobacco smoke has on our health. It is, after all, widely reported. We cannot escape the dreadful consequences of a lifetime of smoking. Cigarette packets, of course, now carry various sickening images such as a child exhaling smoke and, in particular, a man with a huge cancerous growth on his neck. Have you seen that one? I'm sure you have seen them all.

But perhaps the most talked about and terrifying smoking-related disease is, to my mind, lung cancer. The mere notion of it frightened me as a smoker and, to be honest, frightens me still. There are statistics galore out there that will tell you that most lung cancer cases are caused by smoking. Be in no doubt that smoking is its primary cause. As it stands, as a smoker you are considerably more likely to die from lung cancer than someone who has never smoked, and evidence is now suggesting that the younger you start, the greater the risk of permanent lung damage.

There are two main types of the disease: non-small cell lung cancer (NSCLC) and small cell lung cancer (SCLC), but there are many sub-types. The most common form of lung cancer is NSCLC. SCLC is the least common of the two but spreads faster and can grow more quickly. Non-smokers very rarely get SCLC. The survival rates for lung cancer are sadly not high. The chances are that lung cancer will kill you. Early symptoms can be a chronic cough, weight loss, breathlessness and fatigue, among other things – many symptoms smokers are used to, in fact, hence why many cases are detected too late. Imagine for a moment you were told you had lung cancer, that it was growing in your lung uncontrollably. Would smoking seem worth it then?

One of the best things about quitting smoking is the removal of that fear for my health and, ultimately, my life. Every little pain, every twinge was, I believed, the onset of lung cancer or something equally nasty. I'm not saying that quitting smoking guarantees good health, but what it does do is put you back in the driving seat. Every day that passes sees the chances of your contracting an awful disease diminish.

I remember, years ago, being invited to a wedding reception. The bride was a middle-aged woman whom I didn't know and spoke to only briefly. At some point during the night the friend who had invited me told me something that chilled me to the bone. The bride was, he said gravely, dying of lung cancer. She only expected to live a matter of months and had rushed through the wedding plans lest it be left too late.

Can you imagine that? Trying to enjoy what is one of the most special days of your life knowing you will soon be dead? I can't. What was worse, the bride and nearly every other guest were puffing away like chimney towers in a dystopian cityscape. I was too, naturally. The whole room was enveloped in acrid smoke. Knowing the tragedy that underscored the event, you would think many guests would think twice about smoking. But no. They were addicts who had to smoke, even when presented with such a vividly grim reminder of their own mortality. Such is the mind of a smoker.

Lung cancer of course is synonymous with smoking, yet there is a glut of other cancers that are more common in smokers than in non-smokers, including bladder, nose, mouth, larynx, pancreas and many more. Imagine been told you had any of those. You would be terrified. I know I would be. But what would be just as bad would be the knowledge that you could have prevented it, that you could still be healthy and hopeful instead of facing the blankness of death.

Don't go on kidding yourself.

Lung cancer is far from alone. The biggest killer currently in the UK is heart and circulatory disease. Your poor heart and circulatory system really are being put through the mill by your addiction. Your heart is the workhorse of the human body, forever pumping blood around our network of veins and arteries to keep us alive. The stress we put it under by smoking is criminal.

For one thing, the carbon monoxide in cigarettes means less oxygen is reaching your heart. Not only that, but smoking causes your heart to work harder (as if it isn't working hard enough already), increasing your blood pressure. And the arteries through which that blood courses are likely clogged with fatty materials due to smoke damage, meaning less available space for the blood to pass through. A smoker is also nearly twice more likely to have a heart attack than a non-smoker. It is a miracle of human design that our bodies are still functioning after so much abuse.

When you think about how central our heart is to our survival, it is amazing that smokers will run the risk of damaging it for the sake of cigarettes. It shows us how far down the line we are in our addiction that the prospect of a heart attack or stroke doesn't put us off smoking. As a smoker, you are considerably more likely to have a heart attack than a lifelong non-smoker. By simply quitting smoking the odds of avoiding such a fate would begin to rise. But we don't quit. We carry on puffing away, pretending we don't care and that all these studies and statistics mean nothing.

The list of diseases goes on and on: emphysema, liver cancer, periodontitis, abdominal aneurysms, bronchitis. Need I go on? Of course a healthy non-smoker can contract any of these illnesses, but smoking increases your chances by a long way.

Life-threatening diseases aside, there are almost endless health concerns for a smoker. There are many men in the UK, perhaps hundreds of thousands, who are impotent as a result of tobacco smoking. This is because smoking causes atherosclerosis, the building-up of fatty deposits in artery walls, which, in turn, decrease blood flow to the penis. So not only does our old chum tobacco lead us closer to a bunch of incurable illnesses, it ruins our sex life, too.

And not just for the men. The ladies, I'm sorry to say, fair little better. Smoking can potentially cause periods to be sore and irregular, as well as possibly invite an early menopause. The early menopause may be caused by low oestrogen levels, which can also bring on diseases such as osteoporosis. And as with male impotence, because smoking reduces blood flow, there is a strong possibility that sexual pleasure is reduced.

As any smoker will know through bitter experience, colds and flu are made considerably worse by smoking. How many times have you had flu or a chest or throat infection and continued to smoke, even though doing so is highly uncomfortable? I remember having a bad case of tonsillitis where I could barely speak. But still I tried to smoke. Because my wife had warned me not to smoke, I sneaked into the garden for a crafty cigarette only for her to discover me. I will never forget the look of bafflement and disappointment on her face as I stood there in the cold, shivering, taking furtive drags and coughing wildly. She must have thought I was mad.

But it is the day-to-day effects of smoking that I am glad to have left behind for good: the stained teeth and tongue, the bad breath, the tight chest, the hacking cough. Since quitting all these things have improved. When you are a smoker you don't realize how far down smoking has dragged you. I lie in bed at night now and my breathing doesn't have a ragged edge to it any more. I snore less, too, or so I'm told. I still get out of breath, but my breathing seems more controlled now.

As a smoker, you will be aware of how little energy you have and how minor physical challenges are a source of great difficulty. As a smoker, walking up the stairs was a shattering affair, and anything that involved running would leave me on the verge of vomiting. I used to enjoy playing football as a youngster, as well as forever scrambling up trees. Two decades on and I was wheezing like an old horse. What had I done? How could I have slipped this far?

Smokers don't care much for sporty activity. Not only are they usually not up to it, but a sustained period of exercise will interfere with their smoking. Smoking and exercise. Never were two undertakings so diametrically opposed. There are virtually no professional sportspeople out there who smoke. The very idea would put an end to their careers. Even sports like snooker and darts, which have a long association with tobacco through advertising and require little in the way of athletic fitness, have moved away from this smoke-ridden image. No sporting body wants *that* association.

How many times have you slid out of bed in the morning after a night of heavy smoking with a tight, mucus-filled chest? As smokers we go through life in this sluggish manner, our breathing shallow, pains in our abdomen, a constant tickly cough. As a smoker my nose was permanently blocked. When I slept at night I would make an awful gurgling sound, like someone throttling a chicken.

Once you are free of tobacco your body will begin to heal. This will take time. I won't fill you with false hope. You won't begin leaping out of bed every morning and doing a half-marathon before breakfast. You won't suddenly feel like a superhero. Your recovery will happen slowly but surely. There will be days when you feel rough. Embrace these times and remember your health is on its way home.

Another thing that bothered me as a smoker was the idea of premature ageing. I have never been overly concerned with my looks but the idea that smoking would likely add several years to my apparent age and render my face a roadmap of wrinkles was somewhat worrying. To be honest, I didn't need a scientific report to tell me that smokers look older and wrinklier than non-smokers. You will know this yourself. I can almost tell a smoker from a non-smoker just by looking. Smokers seem to have considerably more wrinkles, most obviously around the eyes. Smokers also seem to have a slightly ghost-like appearance, a milky look to the eyes and a grayness of the face.

Don't be in any doubt about the effect tobacco smoke has on your skin. For one thing, smoking causes your skin to break down by reducing the blood flow to the dermis, meaning the outer layer of skin becomes less pliant and able to cope with day-to-day stresses. Cigarette smoke can also cause an over-production of the enzyme matrix metalloproteinase, which is responsible for breaking down skin by inhibiting the creation of fresh collagen. Moreover, smoking reducing our levels of vitamins A and C, both of which help maintain our precious skin. There is even a suggestion that the act of dragging on a cigarette repeatedly contributes to our skin's premature wrinkling.

As a smoker you cannot escape the detrimental effects to your looks. Even if your skin remains relatively youthful-looking, there are still the yellow teeth and fingers, not to mention the permanent odour of stale tobacco. But smokers will turn a blind eye to these things – another example of the addicted mind at work. We will accept a life of staining and ill-health and premature ageing if it means the continuation of our addiction. Such is the madness of smoking.

You see, our fooled brain is telling us that smoking is essential because the nicotine is releasing dopamine, our reward for a job well done. Get this clear in your mind: *Breathing in smoke is not a pleasurable thing to do. If it was, we would loiter around bonfires trying to get a fix or wrap our lips around a car's exhaust pipe in desperate times. It is the nicotine, sending false yet convincing messages, that is tricking you into believing smoking is pleasurable and rewarding. It is as simple as that.*

I'm not trying to scare you by painting a bleak picture of the fate of a smoker. But as I have said, the only way to break free from tobacco is to know it intimately – and that includes its dangers. You can't go through life pretending the hazards don't exist. Of course, life-long non-smokers can fall victim to lung cancer, too, but the chances are slim. Smoking will increase your odds considerably. It is time to face up to reality. The future is not a make-believe place, a far off fantasy. It is real and it is coming your way. How many times have you said you will quit when you're ready? I know I said it hundreds of times. But eventually I did quit. If you desire freedom, then sooner or later you will have to quit too.

Don't leave it till it's too late.

10. The 'Benefits' of Smoking

'I love smoking. How I wish it would love me back.'

~Anonymous

IN 1950 AN EPIDEMIOLOGIST named Richard Doll under-took an in-depth study of lung cancer sufferers and arrived tortuously at the conclusion that smoking tobacco was the root cause of his patients' shared disease. So convinced was Doll of his findings that he even gave up smoking himself. From this point onwards, study after study has shown that smoking tobacco is exceptionally dangerous to human health. We now live in an age in which there is no doubt about tobacco's injurious effect to our health. Yet still a large portion of humanity continues to smoke.

Surely, if so many smoke then there has to be a few plus points to smoking. Surely smoking must have its advantages, however small. After all, there could be the best part of 2 billion smokers worldwide. Surely they must be getting something from it. The idea of positives and advantages justifying smoking is, as you will see, quite ridiculous. I used to think smoking was essential. I couldn't imagine how I would live without it. How would I cope with stress? How would I do anything even slightly taxing without a faithful cigarette to fortify my nerves? When I quit for good, I learned that these worries were unfounded and nothing more than excuses to smoke – attempts to rationalize the irrational. You too would probably reel off a list of smoking's attributes if challenged about your addiction.

Each and every time you have rationalized smoking you have had no choice but to do so. You are an addict, don't forget. You must smoke. Which means you must employ spurious logic and phony arguments to keep the wolves from the door. Deep down, you know you can't justify smoking, but you must manufacture these reasons to smoke lest you are forced to quit.

Smoking relieves stress. That is the common axiom. Like I pointed out earlier, tobacco companies, movies and media in general have sold us this image, and gone on reinforcing it. As a smoker, when you smoke you feel better, right? A cigarette calms you down and helps you put things into perspective. Well actually, yes it does − to a point. But only because the cigarette is responsible for causing that stress in the first place. Remember nicotine's elimination half-life? As the alkaloid is absorbed by your bloodstream its effects wear off − quickly. This makes you feel itchy and unsettled and, through the conditioning, creates a feeling of 'I need a fag.'

But you wouldn't have felt that way, your brain wouldn't have issued such an edict, had you not smoked the last cigarette, which placed nicotine into your body. Do you see the cycle? You are setting yourself up for a life of stress. And what happens when you experience real stress? You smoke like a chimney − only nicotine can't relieve the real stress, only the counterfeit chemical stress of nicotine withdrawal. Next time you feel stress and smoke to relieve it, stop and think. Notice how the cigarette only removes the withdrawal symptoms briefly and how the genuine stress is still there.

Cigarettes really do contain properties that can calm you down. The dopamine you receive creates a sense of satisfaction whilst the beta-endorphin has a relaxing effect. But does that mean you need to inhale carcinogenic smoke to feel this way? Of course not. A drink and sit down can do that. Do you really want to run the risk of lung cancer and heart disease, of impotence and arthritis, just to relax briefly? No, you don't – but that's what you're doing.

You need to start seeing the cigarette in its true light. It is nothing more than dried, finely chopped leaves in a tube of thin paper that you set fire to and inhale. Within the chopped leaves is an alkaloid called nicotine, which after a while will see you addicted to those vile fumes. There is no stress relief whatsoever. It is only the withdrawal from nicotine, which feels a little like stress, that is momentarily reduced. It is just a chemically-induced trick. If you want to avoid a feeling of stress then stop smoking.

Nicotine is a psychoactive drug. In other words, it passes the blood brain barrier and directly affects the central nervous system. Psychoactive drugs are separated into three categories: stimulants, depressants and hallucinogens. Nicotine, it appears, falls into two of these groups, acting as both a depressant and stimulant and certain times. So does this mean, then, that nicotine has positive effects, and that if you are prepared to run the gauntlet of diseases and ill health there are good things to be gained?

I think this is where our twisted perception of cigarettes and smoking comes into play. Imagine someone invented a medicinal inhaler that, when taken, could give you a slight boost while also having relaxing qualities. Imagine this inhaler also partially suppressed your appetite and seemed to relieve stress, if only temporarily. That would be a good thing, wouldn't it? A very useful aid.

But then you learn about the bad side. Apparently, once you start using the inhaler you will become hopelessly addicted to it, having to take a hundred or so puffs a day to keep the feeling going. And then you discover it is dangerous. It can cause lung cancer and heart disease; it will clog your arteries and cause angina and arthritis; it will destroy your fitness and prematurely age your skin; it will stain your teeth and fingers. And then you learn, as if it wasn't already bad enough, that it costs a small fortune to take regularly. And to cap it all off, it actually causes the stress that it is supposed to relieve. Tell me honestly, would you be rushing out to stock up on these things?

No, no and no. But that is what you are doing when you smoke. You are smoking because you are addicted to nicotine, to the feeling a cigarette produces. All these supposed positive feelings are mainly just the result of satisfying your cravings, of ending the restlessness of not being able to smoke. If you were not a smoker then you wouldn't be suffering these effects. Do you see how it works? It is a clever trick and you have been duped.

There is apparently evidence out there that smoking can affect your mood positively, such as increasing concentration and memory and giving you a feeling of stimulus. Well, nicotine is a stimulant, after all. While nicotine's supposed relaxing properties are likely down to the relieving of cravings and resultant endorphin release, the stimulus you receive is highly effective. Nicotine causes a release of adrenaline and glucose. As such, there is often a feeling of being alert and your metabolism quickens. The boost of adrenaline sends you into 'flight or fight' mode. Dopamine, which, as we already know, stimulates the reward pathway, is let loose. Generally speaking, we receive a very real, if temporary, boost.

But so what? We get a similar boost from a coffee or sugary drink. As for adrenaline, our brain releases it when we need it. Why inhale toxic fumes for the effect? Why invite the possibility of numerous cancers into your life? We do it because smoking has its feet under the table; our minds have been warped to except it as something beneficial. It isn't. A quick boost isn't worth your life, is it? You need to move away from these ideas that smoking is serving you well in some way. It isn't. Most of a cigarette's apparent qualities come simply from relieving the craving the cigarette caused. How pointless.

Surely, then, if nothing else, cigarettes improve a night out drinking, or a glass of wine at home. Everybody knows that alcohol and cigarettes go hand-in-hand. But why do we smoke more when drinking? And once we have quit smoking, will a drink ever be the same?

There are a few easily explained reasons as to why our desire for a cigarette seems to increase when we are drinking alcohol. To many smokers a drink without a cigarette is unthinkable. They compliment each other like roast beef and mustard or Ant and Dec. A worry many smokers go through is the thought of ever enjoying a drink again. I can tell you now that there is nothing to worry about.

An alcoholic drink is, of course, something many of us enjoy. We enjoy the effect it gives us. But alcohol has other uses beyond creating an atmosphere of merriment at weddings and wakes. It has medicinal properties, too, one of which is as an anesthetic. And what does anesthetic do? It numbs. Do you remember my mentioning how I would drink tea with a cigarette to lessen the effect? The same goes for alcohol, although booze is much more effective. Instead of just partially blanking the taste of the fag, it actually numbs your mouth, and in doing so lessens the effect of the cigarette. That is why we are able to smoke like a house fire when drinking.

But the numbness is just the beginning. Smoking associations tend to have a field day when alcohol is about. Because we often drink in company – at the pub, at weddings and funerals, at parties – we create a lot of triggers. Talking and socializing isn't stressful, but it takes more brainpower and forethought than when keeping your own company. Talking to others creates subtle tensions and occasions us to share our opinions and listen to others'. This social intercourse can create subtle symptoms similar to nicotine withdrawal and keep us lighting up. And the glut of fellow smokers similarly puffing away only reinforces these triggers. As always, at parties there is a group of smokers congregating in a doorway somewhere, handing out cigarettes and soliciting them. Even if you are on your own, alcohol in your system is enough to heighten your senses and inadvertently create cravings. Alcohol has manufactured a web of strong triggers that you are afraid of defying by quitting. Don't be. It is all in the mind.

I like a drink. I did when I was a smoker, and I do still. I don't binge drink and I'm certainly not an alcoholic, but I enjoy a glass of wine or a beer sometimes and wouldn't change that. But since giving up smoking has drinking become less of a pleasurable experience? Actually, quite the reverse. Since quitting, I enjoy a drink more than ever. Why?

The first reason is down to my stubborn lazy streak. As a smoker, when drinking I found I needed to smoke a lot more. Because of the kids I never smoked in the house, so I was forced, whatever the weather, to disappear into the garden to get my fix. So I found myself on the doorstep every twenty minutes or so, puffing away. When I look back now I realize that having to do this was completely spoiling my evening, not enhancing it. Instead of putting my feet up and relaxing, I constantly had to disappear outside to satisfy my cravings.

I still wake up occasionally with a slight fuzziness in my head if I have had a few drinks the night before. But what is nice is that now my mouth and throat aren't raw and ragged from the endless succession of fags I forced down my neck the night before. When you wake up, you see, the analgesic effects of the alcohol have worn off, leaving your poor throat feeling like you've swallowed a cheese grater.

And when all is said and done, a glass of wine or a beer simply tastes better without the tainted presence of tobacco. Just remember everything you now know about smoking. How can sucking back smoke from burning leaves improve a drink? It can't at all. It is just the relief from the withdrawal of nicotine, an end to the agitation, and your shot of rewarding dopamine that seem to make it pleasurable. But you know it is a scam.

In the next chapter we will deal with the issue of quitting smoking and gaining weight. Many people cite weight gain as a genuine perk to continued tobacco use. Believe me, it isn't. Imagine earlier what I said about the medicinal inhaler, but imagine instead it was a diet pill. You may loose a little weight, but a glut of killer diseases and a lifetime of servitude await you. You wouldn't rush out to buy it, would you? Of course not. But like I said, this issue deserves its own chapter.

But for now let's look into last chance saloon. Okay, so we know smoking is pointless – needless slavery. Any vague and temporary boost is utterly overshadowed by the wealth of deleterious effects to your health and fitness and finances. But surely there is at least one saving grace, a chink of good amid a wealth of bad. Cigarettes clearly will kill us, or at least shorten our lives, but maybe the social graces smoking offers are worth the gamble.

I mean, surely a well-placed cigarette can add a touch of sophistication to a scene, lend a dash of rakish charm. Believe it or not, I believe it can – at least, to a point. I know I said earlier that the cigarette in Audrey Hepburn's holder wasn't sophisticated, but I wanted to make a point about our distorted view of cigarettes. What I don't want to do is airbrush smoking from history like some people and organizations desire to do. It has a place in history. I believe, more so in the West, that we are heading towards an increasingly cigarette-intolerant society. The succession of smoking bans in public places is just the start. Soon cigarettes will be what snuff is today: a strange, old-school drug that seems outmoded in a modern, health-conscious world. One day cigarettes will be illegal, I'm sure.

But that isn't to say tobacco was never there. Certain imagery will always be linked to smoking. Can you imagine Churchill without his trademark cigar? Although I know that cigar is utterly pointless and health-damaging, I still think it belongs there, in *that* place at *that* time. How about those old black-and-white Hollywood films where the leads are sharing a cigarette amid a tearful farewell? I wouldn't change that. Tobacco is too ingrained in our culture to pretend it was never there. Ultimately, I don't want to see smoking taken away from people who genuinely want to keep it. Each to their own.

But it is important that you, as someone who wants to quit, separate a little indulgent sentimentality from a very real and dangerous drug addiction. Don't forget that these people you see smoking, whether on the big screen or on television or in the street, are drug addicts, forced to smoke to get the nicotine and defuse their cravings. There is no inherent glamour or sophistication in a cigarette – that is just imagery. Tobacco smoke is nothing more than chemicals and carcinogens. See it as it is. You now know the trick, so be careful not to keep falling for it.

11. Good Times

'Smoking is hateful to the nose, harmful to the brain, and dangerous to the lungs.'

~King James I of England

TO BE HONEST, I could write a chunky novel-length work on the endless benefits that quitting smoking will bring to your life. The sense of freedom you have to look forward to is unrivaled. Whenever I think about my tobacco addiction now, I see how fortunate I was to have escaped for good. Life without cigarettes is so much better than a life of smoke-stained slavery.

But first I need to share with you a hard truth, a truth that will prepare you for your new smoke-free life. And it is this. When you quit smoking, *nothing will happen.* There will be no fanfare or parade in your honour. After quitting, you won't spring out of bed every morning like an athlete and run a three-minute mile. You won't suddenly be the master of all you survey. The sun will not always shine and you will not be wrapped up in a permanent state of contentment. The reality of quitting smoking is somewhat less exciting. Life will be what it was before, but without the familiarity of tobacco. That's about it.

I'm not telling you all this to knock your confidence. I just want you to enter your new smoke-free life with your feet firmly on the ground and your head out of the clouds. I just want you to know that life won't suddenly be a fairytale. Life isn't perfect whilst you are smoking, so why should it be perfect when you quit? Life, as always, will have its moments of triumph and times of anguish.

Why am I telling you all this? I'm simply preparing you for the reality of quitting. There is in fact another element of psychology at play here. Earlier we looked at how society's wisdom suggests that quitting smoking is hard, when that isn't necessarily the case. Another axiom, another bedrock of truth perpetuated by certain organizations is that once you quit smoking you enter some sort of Promised Land, a utopia of healthfulness and endless sunshine and far-reaching blue skies. I'm sorry, but it isn't like that. This is just anti-smoking establishment propaganda.

The big pharmaceutical companies who make nicotine patches and gum and other cessation products, not to mention the abundance of quit smoking charities and other anti-smoking organizations, need to sell you a pristine image of life without tobacco. Their aim, whether it be financial or simply to justify their own existence, is for you to quit smoking. Therefore, they must advertise. And advertising is about selling imagery. When you watch car adverts on television, why do they always seem to comprise a good-looking man or woman driving along empty, winding country roads with a Mediterranean-style backdrop of blue sea and rich sunlight?

The advertisers paint the experience of driving their cars like this because the actual reality is not a good enough sales point. If we were treated to a more likely image of two stressed parents loading a gaggle of screaming, whining children into the car and then see them sitting in gridlocked rush-hour traffic as torrential rain pounds off the windscreen, such scenes would hardly help sell the car in question, would they? The advertisers only give us falsified scenes of comfort and style because that is what consumers react to. Anti-smoking advertising in no different.

Even the British National Health Service (NHS) depicts in its literature a blessed and content life once cigarettes have been shown the door – newly emancipated smokers standing on grassy hillsides with the sun on their faces, and so on. With all this imagery and suggestion it is small wonder we come to believe there is a life of limitless joy once we're past our addiction. There isn't, I'm afraid. It's just plain old life. Of course, I haven't got anything whatsoever against anti-smoking groups or campaigns, but I want you to see the whole picture clearly. Let's not leave anything to chance.

But that's enough grimness now. I hope I haven't depressed you too much. I just feel it has been necessary to illustrate life after smoking so frankly to avoid a sense of anti-climax on your part. I don't want you to quit with false expectations, that's all. That is not to say life isn't sweet as a non-smoker. It is, believe me. I would never go back to those days of choking myself, of waking up with a clogged chest and coughing away constantly.

The truth is that you will start to feel better almost straightaway once you have quit smoking. It is a long and winding road back to your former days of smoke-free health, but the time will fly by and you will get there eventually. Within a short amount of time you should notice your breathing begin to get better. I found my ability to take in air improve almost immediately, although I should say that even now it isn't like it was. That will take time. But I know I will get there.

A hacking cough might develop, but don't worry about

that – it is part of the healing process. Our lower respiratory tracts are lined with minute hairs called cilia, which act like sweepers, moving unwanted debris out of our bodies. Tobacco smoke kills off these tiny cilia. Once you stop smoking, however, they will once again begin in earnest doing their job, hence the cough as the cilia expel the residual tar and other nasty things. Go with it and don't worry.

For a while you might well feel worse than you did as a smoker. Your body is going through a harsh regime change. I remember feeling somewhat odd for a few days after quitting. But I knew the rough ride was all part of the healing process. For years I had been wantonly pumping my body full of toxins. And suddenly I pulled the plug. This new routine will take time to adjust to. You might feel lightheaded, too. This is the life-preserving oxygen in your bloodstream replacing the carbon monoxide that has been a regular feature for as long as you have smoked. Whatever strange and disagreeable sensations you have, stay positive and revel in the fact you have begun the process of recovery.

Smoking has had an affect on your appearance, too, whether you can accept this or not. The good news is that a lot of these effects are reversible. Those ugly yellow stains on your fingers will go in time, and so will that yellow sheen to your teeth. Like I have already remarked, I drank a lot of tea and coffee whilst smoking. Fewer cups have no doubt helped my teeth whiten. I often look in the mirror and glory at my new twinkling game show-host smile (well, almost).

One of the greatest indignities of smoking is that we must fund it. Cigarettes seem to rise dramatically in price with each passing year. We all know that agonized sense of self-loathing as we hand over an obscene amount of money for our cigarettes – in the knowledge that they will not last long and we will soon be back for more.

I used to feel at my most stupid and addicted when it came to the monetary side of smoking. As rational human beings, we know the idea of paying dearly for a substance that is destroying our health and fitness is crass and contrary to any logic, yet our addicted brain needs its fix. So we must acquiesce. I used to hate myself for wasting money on tobacco. Having young children just made it even worse.

At some point many years ago I switched to rolling tobacco during a period of financial moderation (I was broke, in other words). If I was going to poison myself and destroy my health and fitness, the least I could do was pay as little as possible for it. And I'm sure I did make some sort of saving by switching. But that isn't the point, is it? Why pay anything? Why smoke at all? During the last years of smoking I didn't even pretend to like doing it and resented the loss of money more than ever.

Let's be honest. Most of us work hard and can afford to smoke, more or less. Of course we would be better off not smoking, but we manage, don't we? But that is just not the point. The point is that we are needlessly poisoning ourselves, sucking back the fumes from dried leaves over and over and over again because we think we enjoy it. That is the core stupidity of smoking. That we pay for it is just a further insult to add to the pile. If you want to break free from smoking then you must focus your thoughts correctly. Being better off money-wise is another advantage of quitting, but we must see that smoking is a futile, pointless exercise and that we never needed to do it. Think of the freedom that awaits you.

*

Like I said earlier, the benefits of quitting smoking could probably fill endless pages. In good time your health will improve. You will be fitter and healthier and certainly look better. You will have more money in your pocket. You will be ready to deal with life without the black cloud of smoking hanging over you.

But all of these things pale into insignificance when compared to quitting smoking's greatest gift. The gift of yourself. For as long as you have been a smoker you have been a prisoner, confined to a cell of your own making. Do you even remember what it is like to be a non-smoker? Nicotine has for too long controlled those dopamine pathways, making you a slave, forcing you to breathe in poisonous fumes to get your next fix. Everything you have experienced in life has been conditional on topping up your ailing levels of nicotine, day in, day out. When I was deprived of cigarettes, for even a short time, I could think of little else. It invades your mind and ruins moments of your life that should be special.

I was seventeen when I first went on a plane. For years I had waited to experience the sensation of soaring above the clouds and seeing the world below in miniature. It should have been a wonderful, memorable moment. Once in the sky, I remember only vaguely an endless vista of sea and mountains, a blood-red sun sinking in a haze of gold. But I was restless and not really concentrating. All I could think was, 'How long now? I'm gasping for a fag!' My maiden journey on a plane ended up being nothing more than an obstacle to smoking. Do you see how nicotine addiction robs you of moments that should be precious?

When you quit smoking, slowly, without your really noticing, you start to return to your former self, the person you were before you got yourself hijacked by tobacco. Simple things, the little things, seem important and worthwhile. Ever since quitting I have had a subtle, underlying sense of happiness; nothing special, just a quiet feeling of contentment. And I know that returning to smoking would see an end to this state of mind. I still suffer stress. I still have times when I am unhappy. But I never forget that I now have the superlative advantage of not being addicted to smoking anymore. It is a great feeling to be free.

You have this to look forward to.

12. Eat and Be Merry

'Stained teeth, bad breath and black lungs are worth it to avoid the curse of fat thighs.'

~Anonymous

'IF I QUIT SMOKING I'LL blow up like a balloon.'

The idea of putting on weight is, as you will probably know, one of the most oft-cited reasons for returning to smoking or, equally, not bothering to quit in the first place. The truth is, espousing your concerns about piling on the flesh and then using them as a justification to continue to smoke is not, by a long way, a good enough basis to persist in your addiction. Like all other aspects of quitting smoking, the weight issue is a matter of perspective.

Let's be brutally honest here. When we quit smoking many of us tend to put on a little weight. Why bother to gloss over the truth? I have spoken to a lot of smokers about weight gain and the consensus is that, yes, after quitting smoking a few surplus pounds tend to creep on. In most cases nothing more than a few rogue pounds find their way onto your hips or thighs or stomach. Nothing much else. Of course, there are those of you that will indeed blow up like balloons. If you eat frequently and greedily then naturally obesity is on the cards. Your food intake, remember, is in your hands. But ceasing to breathe in tobacco smoke is not alone going to cause you to gain weight.

It is true, however, that tobacco seems to serve as an

appetite suppressant, and has been used historically as such. The tobacco companies have in the past played up to the notion that smoking keeps you slim. In the late 1920s there was a cigarette brand called Lucky Strike that marketed its cigarettes towards women as a way of controlling the appetite and thus keeping trim. Lucky Strike, as a result of the campaign, became a runaway success.

Tobacco smoke, as you know, decreases your sensitivity to taste, meaning food doesn't seem quite as tasty to smokers. One of the things I have noticed since quitting is that food appears to have considerably more taste. Subtle flavours are now zingier. Watercress, which as a smoker tasted to me completely plain, now presents a pleasant earthy flavour. And if food is more pleasant to eat then I suppose it follows logically that you will consume it in heartier portions.

Furthermore, and on a somewhat obvious note, if you are puffing away on a cigarette then you are probably not eating. I used to find that I would not eat for hours at a time because of smoking, often skipping meals. I hated the combination of tobacco smoke and food and kept them distinctly separate. There is simply no doubt in my mind that your smoking addiction means an ultimately smaller food intake.

In truth, every time I have quit smoking the weight has crept on, often with alarming speed. I've come across many people who have gone back to smoking simply to avoid any more fleshing out. Is a future of obesity – or at least struggling with our weight – simply a cross we must bear if we're to quit smoking and never go back? The answer isn't straightforward, I'm afraid. I'm not going to make any pointless promises about your future as a non-smoker. I haven't so far and I won't start now. If – like me – you have racked up a number of failed attempts at quitting then you'll know that weight gain is a very real issue. You might, of course, be one of those lucky souls who don't gain anything and might rightly be wondering what all the fuss is about. For those of you in this enviable position it is simply one less thing for you to consider when quitting. For the rest of us mere mortals, we need a workable strategy.

The first and most important thing I want to point out about weight gain is that it is not the end of the world. So what if, for a while, you fill out? Remember that you are purging an evil, health-damaging drug addiction from your life. You are compelled at present to breathe in a noxious, eye-watering mixture of poisonous gases in the false belief that you are receiving something beneficial and essential. If I gave you a choice of the two following options, which would you choose? Option one: gain a few pounds, perhaps a stone, which you can always lose through exercise and healthy eating. Option two: spend the rest of your life being forced to breath in a cocktail of injurious fumes in the mistaken belief that they are benefitting you, when actually they're killing you. So, what would it be? When laid out candidly like that, it's a no brainer, isn't it?

Stop smoking!

It is time to make some hard yet vital choices. You have to ask yourself just how much you want to quit tobacco smoking, how much you desire to see the back of it for good. The answer, unequivocally, should be 'Yes! I desperately want this, more than anything.' If you genuinely feel that way, then gaining weight shouldn't be such a depressing and all-consuming issue. Surely your life is worth more than a few rogue pounds of flesh. The only exception I would make is if you are already dangerously overweight and further weight-gain could be life-threatening. In this case, you need to consult your doctor. My advice, I truly believe, will still help you to quit smoking, but only when it is safe for you to do so – so to speak.

If you really want to wave goodbye to smoking then it is time to get philosophical. You are a drug addict. The drug you are beholden to is a killer. Even if you avoid one of the horrendous illnesses, you face a life of gunged-up tobacco consumption, a life of zero energy and get-up-and-go. A life of breathless aversion to physical activity. By continuing to puff away you will shorten your time on this earth almost certainly. Ask yourself: will a few pounds really matter? Is gaining a little weight any sort of justification to continue to smoke. The answer is *no, of course not!*

What we have here is typical drug addict thinking. Any excuse to continue to use. A little weight gain is, in your twisted book, enough justification to go on puffing away. Do you see? Don't even let the issue of weight-gain show on your radar. Don't turn it into a big deal. All you should be thinking about is your new smoke-free life, a life of energy, a life freed from the claws of chemical addiction. Because that is all smoking is: addiction to a chemical, the alkaloid nicotine. Be positive and focus on the future. In truth, you will probably be pleasantly surprised by how little your weight alters. But if you do bulk-out somewhat, stay calm and bear in mind the huge bonus of *no more cigarettes.*

Once you've stopped smoking, your body will, like I have said, be in turmoil for a while. That is all part of the healing process. Once your lungs have recovered from smoking, you'll be markedly more able to exercise than you are currently able to. Your energy levels will, after time, improve. You will feel healthier and doubtless possess an underlying sense of positivity, which will encourage you into exercise.

Any weight you've initially gained will be easily burned away as you rediscover a healthier new you. Don't get me wrong. I'm not trying to paint a fairytale here. Some of you might simply not be cut out for sportiness and will struggle to shift that stubborn flesh. I don't exercise much more than I did before, but I feel possessed of a streak of energy that I lacked as a smoker. I'm no athlete. But I feel so much healthier. Remember, you are going to rid yourself of an awful chemical addiction that is destroying you. Be positive.

This is about quitting smoking, not quitting life. You don't have to become some lettuce munching, carrot juice-drinking yoga nut. You will still be you. I eat some pretty bad foods at times and enjoy a beer or a glass of wine. I have accepted now that I will never be a health freak. But always, flirting at the fringes of my conscience, is the brilliant truth that smoking is no longer the master of my life.

13. Attitude Is Everything

'Much smoking kills live men and cures dead swine.'

~George D. Prentice

WHEN WE ATTEMPT TO QUIT smoking our attitude plays a crucial role. In fact, *attitude is everything*. It is paramount. Approaching quitting smoking with the correct mind-set will not only prepare you for your new smoke-free life but will prevent you going back. I have learned how to shape my attitude through years of failed attempts to quit. Even now I have to keep certain philosophies intact, making sure I'm seeing smoking as it really is. But after time keeping this correct attitude becomes second nature.

Simply put, it is our attitude to smoking that keeps us hooked. Of course, nicotine takes care of the physical side of things, but the real barrier is our own web of misapprehensions; we are, in essence, both the jailor and the jailed. Our poor minds have been conditioned through years of smoking to believe our next fix of nicotine is all-important – essential to our survival and well-being. Our brain might be a complex supercomputer, but tobacco has managed to fool it into thinking smoking is vital for life. In truth smoking is the absolute polar opposite.

When we are deprived of our precious cigarettes our conditioned brain generates a craving, which we are forced to answer. Only smoking, it seems, can assuage this uneasy feeling, this itchiness. So it is little wonder we have developed a close and personal affection for cigarettes.

They seem irreplaceable, don't they? We know the dangers, but, well … we just need them. They are dangerous but necessary. The friend we can't live with yet can't live without. The truth is you can live without cigarettes, leading a more fulfilled and healthy life. Billions live without tobacco and never feel the need to breathe in those noxious fumes. I'm so glad I am one of these people. You too can be among their ranks soon enough.

We approach quitting smoking with a sense of fear and trepidation. We believe we are entering a dark and unpleasant unknown. We assume we are about to deprive ourselves of something we enjoy: our old chum, our reliable pal. Once we have taken the plunge and stopped smoking, that romantic image of smoking – that rosy view that puts tobacco on a pedestal – takes on a life of its very own. It becomes simply intolerable, this quitting business. At some point we accept that quitting smoking is just too hard, that now is absolutely not the right time. Then we crawl back to tobacco, depressed yet relieved.

We effect this regretful return to smoking because we have not gone about quitting with the right attitude. Had we have had the correct mind-set we would not have felt such a keen sense of loss. But as it is we are forced, through physical addiction and psychological dependency, to go back to smoking for the sake of our own sanity. Does this sound familiar? For many years it was the story of my life.

To possess yourself of the right attitude and keep it intact you need to adjust your view of smoking. Doing so is actually pretty easy if you truly open your mind and discard the old ways. It is sometimes hard to let go of long-held beliefs, but let go you must if you are to be successful. Imagine that you have a pet cat, a male. You have had this cat for years; it is a member of the family. It has its own unique personality. Imagine that you take it to the vets for a jab and the vet notices the cat is in fact female. This would be a shock, right? How did you miss it? It would mean you would have to adjust your view of your pet and put aside everything you thought you knew. But you would, in the end. It might take a little getting used to, but in time you would. You wouldn't continue to see the cat as male. Why would you choose to live in such ignorance?

It is no different with smoking. You have learnt to view it in a certain light. But you can't anymore. You now know you are the victim of a simple yet effective trick. Breathing the fumes from smoldering tobacco isn't essential for life or in any way pleasurable – it is awful. You are now in possession of the truth. You know nicotine releases dopamine, which, in turn, creates the illusion of satisfaction. You need to keep the truth alive in your mind and never let it go.

The idea that a cigarette is in some way rewarding is a con trick. Chemicals are released that tell us we have done the right thing by smoking and that we are feeling good. In a purely scientific sense, we are. But it is a trick, remember, a clever, subtle, invidious confidence trick. How can breathing in a blend of deadly chemicals be what we need, what your body needs for continued well-being? Think about it hard for a moment. Think hard. Is breathing in the fumes from burning tobacco leaves really a good experience? Is poisoning ourselves a good experience? Of course not.

Start from now to see cigarettes as they really are: a life-damaging drug, to which you are addicted. Strip away the appendages, the extras that come with smoking. The gold lighters and scallop shell ashtrays are nothing but the manifestation of a highly addictive and dangerous drug addiction. The respectable, slick face of chemical enslavement. You are an addict and your addiction will kill you or, at the very least, shorten your life. There is nothing sophisticated, nothing trendy and certainly nothing agreeable about tobacco addiction. All you get for your hard-earned cash is a vague delusion of happiness and restfulness and a virtually endless list of killer illnesses.

You must understand smoking fully. The penny must drop. I know it isn't easy. Surely, somewhere, somehow, there must be an upside to smoking. There isn't, not when you look closely. You smoke because you feel itchy and irritable, but it is your nicotine addiction causing those feelings of agitation. It is a pointless, deadly cycle. Cast your mind back to the mists of your childhood. Think about before you started smoking. Do you remember feeling back then as though there was something missing, like your entire life so far was gearing up to discovering some drug to complete your peace of mind? No. You were happy and healthy and complete. Only, you introduced nicotine into the equation. You fooled your complete mind that somehow it needed nicotine. And here you are, all these years later, your mind still the dupe of tobacco. But not for much longer.

From hereon in, see smoking as it really is: dried leaves in a paper tube, to which you set fire and inhale the fumes. Those fumes contain an alkaloid called nicotine that will keep you dependant for life. Unless you break the cycle. By training your mind to see only the truth you will soon lose your desire to keep lighting up. Your mind is more powerful than the cigarette. Don't forget that.

14. Reasoning

'Smoking is one of the leading causes of statistics.'

~Fletcher Knebel

WHEN IT COMES TO quitting smoking, a common prelude to failure can be your motives. Exactly why are you quitting, and for whom? What is driving you to abandon smoking forever? Provided you are giving up for the right reasons, then quitting does not have to be a struggle – in fact it is pretty easygoing. Sound and solid reasoning is what drives you towards quitting and keeps you there. Get that reasoning muddled and misplaced, however, and you will make life very difficult for yourself.

Probably the most common reason for quitting is health. And it isn't surprising, is it? Study after study shows that smoking is exceptionally bad for our health. Millions of people every year are being added to tobacco's death list. Don't be in any doubt: smoking really does kill, and in alarmingly robust numbers. Smokers generally tend to live a life of denial, a life of turning the other cheek, but will occasionally take a peek at the reality of smoking and grow wholly terrified of what they see.

We spend our smoking lives petrified of these health risks yet unable to quit. I know I did. Eventually we decide enough is enough and throw away our cigarettes before our life is claimed by one of the many deadly illnesses associated with smoking. As for which one, take your pick. But why can't we stay away from smoking for good? Why do we go back? Surely the prospect of cancer or heart disease is enough to convince us not to smoke, isn't it? But no. If that were the case, the world would be virtually smoke-free. Health scares have never been sufficient to get us off the cigarettes.

Remember, we smoke because we are addicted to nicotine and psychologically dependant on tobacco. We get a feeling of satisfaction and reward every time we light up. We believe we are receiving something essential to our survival. But what we actually receive is quite the reverse. We know only too well that smoking might kill us – it will almost certainly knock years off our life – but we also harbour the idea that smoking is too precious to relinquish. So we smoke and smoke, ignoring the warnings and flying in the face of common sense and logic.

Money is another worry for the embattled smoker. It's no surprise considering the cost of tobacco. Every year the tax on cigarettes rises dramatically. I remember many people saying that once a twenty-pack reached £5.00 they would quit. Well, five pounds is but a distant memory and those people are still smoking to my knowledge. The truth is, no matter how expensive smoking becomes the fooled smoker will find the money for it – just as they would for food. Your finances might dictate you smoke less, but you will still smoke – you will doubtless beg, steal and borrow to continue to puff away. How many times have you tried to budget your cigarettes, to make them last longer. That never works for too long.

As long as you are convinced that you must smoke, that tobacco is your true friend, you will never quit for good. You are an addict; you are utterly dependent on cigarettes. At the moment you might be able to afford to smoke, but come a time of financial restraint your addiction will not go away. It is at these times that the really ugly part of the addiction comes to the surface.

You might be forced by another person to quit. Maybe there is a baby on the way and money is tight. Maybe you have met someone you're keen on and he or she is a non-smoker. Trying to quit smoking to please someone else is the road to madness. There is no future in it. It is noble, yes – but not realistic. You are an addict, remember. You smoke knowing you could get lung cancer or heart disease, but that hasn't put you off. So why should a polite request from a loved one do the trick? You might hold out for a while, but eventually you will have to smoke lest you go mad.

I remember my wife constantly asking me to quit whilst pregnant with both of our children. I stopped for a very short while but as soon as I could I lit up, often smoking in secret. After our daughter was born my wife said she'd read an article about how tobacco smoke on clothes could make babies ill. She said I should quit, and now, for the sake of our child's health. Can you imagine the panic I experienced? She was trying to take away my precious cigarettes. I told her that the article was a load of old rubbish and continued to smoke.

Now think about the situation. I was just told that smoking could harm our newborn daughter, an infinitely precious person to us. Even if I was completely right and the article was indeed rubbish (which is unlikely), why take the risk? I should have quit there and then just to play it safe. But I didn't. And I will tell you why. Because even then, faced with the prospect of harming my baby's tender lungs, I couldn't bear the thought of not smoking. Cigarettes were just too prized, too much part of me. To compromise, however, I started changing my clothes completely after every cigarette and scrubbing myself down before going near our baby. Enough said.

What I'm trying to say is that there is only one true reason to quit. I could list a million reasons to quit smoking, each one valid, but there is no point. You probably know most of them anyway. The only genuine reason you need to quit smoking is that you *do not want to smoke anymore*. That you understand your addiction inside out and are prepared to purge it from your life forever. With knowledge comes power, and soon you will be in a position to turn the tables on nicotine once and for all.

Money and health and fitness are all fantastic by-products of quitting smoking, but you don't need to make quitting about these things. Knowing how you have been tricked by cigarettes is reason enough to quit. If you feel you will miss smoking and are quitting purely to save money, at some point you will go crawling back to the addiction. The belief that smoking is precious will keep you imprisoned for life unless you take a positive stride towards freedom and finally see the truth.

You can do it.

15. The Time is Right

'My smoking might be bothering you, but it's killing me.'

~Colette

AS I HAVE ALREADY said, quitting smoking doesn't have to be the minefield society has painted it to be. As long as you fully understand your addiction and possess the correct attitude, nothing can prevent you stopping smoking and never going back. But you need the right preparation to succeed. And one of the most crucial factors to your success will not just be *how* or *why* you quit, but *when* you quit

Choosing a poor time to quit smoking is one of the most common reasons for a quick relapse. Rushing headlong into quitting may seem desirable – and is even admirable – but in the long-term it will prove foolhardy and ultimately serve as your downfall. Imagine you are locked in a prison. Rushing like a bull towards the briefly open gate in a bid for freedom might seem quick and easy, but your captors can see you coming and you are always stopped. Now imagine laying careful plans, running through every possibility and leaving nothing to chance. You time your plan to perfection and escape for good. Be patient. Doing so will mean the odds are now stacked in your favour. Timing is everything. Get it right and you will be laughing. Get it wrong and a miserable return to smoking might well be on the cards.

So when is the correct time to quit? Surely if you're serious about quitting then there is no time like the present. That's true, of course – you have been delaying quitting for years. But you are close now. Don't rush. Simply throwing down your cigarettes and pronouncing yourself a non-smoker isn't going to cut the mustard. You might have heard of people doing that – waking up one morning and never smoking again – but such people are rare creatures and I'm willing to bet most of them are exaggerating anyway. Their success was probably limited and at some point they went back to smoking. I know only too well. I've thrown my tobacco in the bin countless times only to find myself fishing it back out within half and hour.

The right time to quit, the optimum time, is during a quiet, routine period of your life, a period of calm and normality. If you attempt to quit during a time of uncertainty and stress then you're heading for a fall. Turmoil in your life is not conducive to quitting, so wait. I'm sorry; I know it's not what you want to hear. But do you want another failed attempt under your belt? Of course you don't. When you quit this time it will be for good – you and tobacco will part company forever. So be patient and wait for the right time. Don't rush; you are nearly there.

The reason you need this subdued and 'normal' period to quit is that during those initial days and weeks familiarity will serve you well. You are used to the smoking triggers of your normal working week. You know them well. You experience them all the time and know when they will arrive. You can twist these moments to your advantage. Whether you are a stay-at-home parent or a full-time worker or presently unemployed, your life will run more or less at a constant. Yes, there might be bumps in the path, but by and large you know what to expect from your day. You know you will crave nicotine in the morning before work. You know once the housework is completed you will want to smoke. You expect these times and can therefore plan for them.

If, for instance, you have a holiday coming up, think carefully before choosing now to quit. Holidays differ from the norm. You may well drink more alcohol than usual and find extra time on your hands. Do you feel confident you can navigate this period without smoking? In truth, I would not attempt it. I'm not saying you couldn't do it; it's just that why choose a tricky time when you can opt for a simple one, right? Wait, just a little longer.

There might, for instance, be a wedding or some other occasion where smoking will be omnipresent. If after that event there is nothing on the horizon, then wait till after it. Why rush? You want to quit smoking and never go back. So be patient. The last you need is to be dealing with strong yet unusual triggers so early on.

When your life returns to normal, then *go for it!*

As you will be acutely aware, smokers tend to smoke like chimney stacks during times of stress. This is because stress feels very much like nicotine withdrawal. Like I have already pointed out, we need our dopamine fix even more when life gets tough – we need, or think we need, the false chemical reassurance that nicotine offers. So we light cigarette after cigarette, burning our throat in the belief we are getting our reward. By now, of course, your immunity to nicotine is going through the roof, so you smoke more and more to achieve an unachievable sense of peace

It is just a trick, a con. Yet trying to quit during such times of agitation is not going to work out. Your head will be all over the place and not on the job. Your focus should be solely on quitting smoking. Stressful moment after stressful moment will carve away your confidence and you will lose faith and eventually smoke. And this time you're not going to do that. This time you will never go back.

But we can't plan our fate, can we? Things will crop up. Life will be sailing along languidly one moment and the next all Hell will break loose. Well, yes. Quite probably. Does that mean you smoke? Of course not. However, if you have quite literally just started out and feel you can't quit because of some unforeseen stress, then listen to your heart. You know yourself. The time will soon be right. But if you are already well into your new smoke-free life then why on earth would you want to go back? A cigarette would taste awful now – absolutely revolting – and do nothing other than pump nicotine back into your system and bring about a full-blown relapse.

Is this what you want? No, of course not!

After I quit smoking my life wasn't magically transformed into a stress-free utopia. Life was the same. My kids were still naughty. I still had to sit in rain-soaked rush hours. I still stubbed my toe at night when visiting the toilet. I still had unexpected bills drop through the letterbox. I still had to deal with all those brain-numbing aspects of modern life. But with one, all-important difference. I wasn't beholden to cigarettes. I wasn't a drug addict, a slave. I was – I am – free.

You will be too.

16. Preparation Mode

'Remember, if you smoke after sex then you're doing it too fast.'

~Woody Allen

THE DAYS AND WEEKS leading up to your final separation from tobacco addiction will be of paramount importance. You might feel presently that you are stuck in a kind of purgatory: wanting to get on with the business of quitting smoking yet holding out for the right moment. That is how I felt and it is actually a good place to be. Patience is essential, yet you should be straining to get on and quit for good.

A sound strategy will ultimately lead to victory over tobacco, and it is during this limbo-like period that you should be planning away. When it comes to quitting for good you can't do half a job. A wishy-washy attitude at this time might prove fatal to your chances of quitting. You should be fortifying your mind, letting all the truisms about tobacco and smoking sink in and solidify into a rock-solid will to kick your addiction into touch, forever. Everything you have learned should have given you an impetus to see the back of smoking. This knowledge will stay with you and protect you from relapse. All you need to do is stay positive and stay focused.

The first step in your plan should be to choose a date to quit. Set this day in stone and work towards it. Look forward to it; it will the first day of your true freedom. Remember to pick a day that will be followed by a period of calm and order. A time of stress and uncertainty will not help you. This is very important. Time that quitting date as close to perfection as possible – you certainly don't want a false start.

Now you have your quitting date, start to gear up towards it. Begin clearing your home of smoking paraphernalia: ashtrays, lighters, tobacco tins. Get rid of these things; give them away or throw them away. You won't need any of them ever again. That precious gold lighter, don't forget, was a tool of your addiction. This is no time for sentimentality. If you must keep anything, put it in a deep, dark drawer and never let it see the light of day. If you find yourself holding on to anything 'just in case', then your attitude needs to change and I would even say you are not ready to quit. Be ruthless with smoking; it has, after all, been utterly ruthless with you.

Don't try to cut down during this time, either. Remember, cutting down just makes tobacco seem more precious. Holding out simply makes the 'relief' of smoking more intense. At this time you really need to start distancing yourself from smoking emotionally, not endearing yourself to it. Besides which, you have probably tried many times to cut down only to find your strategy falling to pieces within days.

If anything – and I give this advice in the earnest belief you will quit – smoke as much as you can during these days and weeks leading up to the big day. Really start to consciously scrutinize every cigarette you smoke. Ask yourself, as you suck the smoke into your lungs, whether you want to have to do this until the day you die – a day that cigarette smoking might well expedite. Take in the smell and taste and realize the truth: it is foul. You smoke so you can get the nicotine and relieve your troubled mind, nothing more.

*

There is one inescapable aspect to quitting smoking that you will have to deal with: cravings. They are inevitable. But remember everything you know about cravings, how we ourselves create them through our false ideologies of smoking. It is simply our approach to cravings that makes it difficult to quit. We tune into them, build them up, make them significant. We buy into our urges to smoke and in doing so make life very tough. But armed with the right attitude, these moments are easily traversed. It is all about how you view the situation. Perception is everything.

For instance, if you make a coffee and suddenly get a strong urge to smoke, why are you surprised? You shouldn't be. Your addicted brain has been commanding you to light up during such moments for years. Just because you've made a *conscious* decision to quit smoking, it doesn't mean your *subconscious* mind will agree with this new direction. It won't. It will expect you to smoke and will throw a tantrum if you deny it its fix. This is why the right attitude, starting *now*, is so crucial.

No longer see cigarettes as your pleasurable vice, your coffee-time companion. Smoking is nothing more than drug addiction that lasts a lifetime unless you make a confident decision to stop the rot. By letting the truth about smoking wash into your subconscious mind you will slowly train it to see smoking as it is: filthy, costly, life-threatening and utterly pointless. Start now. Let these ideas soak in. They will probably save your life.

When you make that coffee, or partake in any activity that will trigger a need to smoke, work through it rationally. Go through the steps I described earlier: abdominal breathing followed by a careful analysis of how you feel. Think about how smoking is doing nothing to help you but a lot to harm you. Think about that noxious smoke cascading down your throat and consider how you have been tricked by the alkaloid nicotine and its lethal delivery system into thinking that this cocktail of deadly chemicals is somehow pleasurable and beneficial. Cast off those blinkers and see it clearly.

By preparing in this way you will lay the foundations of a successful transition from addiction to freedom. A little planning and a little thinking are worth your life, aren't they? Being mentally prepared for quitting smoking is critical to your success. If your head isn't in the right place you will set yourself up for failure. Don't be complacent. Build your fortifications now, not when the enemy is already streaming over the walls.

Don't bother stocking up on nicotine patches and gum and so on. You won't need them. They will complicate things for you. For a while nicotine will be leaving your body. By placing fresh nicotine into your system you will keep the agitation going. Why bother? Likewise pills: the last thing you need is to swap one addiction for another.

I'm not saying I necessarily disagree with cessation products; it is just that they will, I believe, serve as a distraction. If you are really adamant that you want to use a quit-aid, then do so carefully and have a focused plan to wean yourself off it as quickly as possible. As long as you keep in mind the truth about smoking you should be able to quit pretty easily, whether you use these things or not. Just be careful.

You should, by rights, be full of almost child-like enthusiasm at the thought of quitting smoking and never having to go back. If so, you will doubtless be anxious to tell the world and his wife about your imminent lifestyle change. By all means do so – but be careful. Whilst nothing should stand in your way, telling too many people can mean you are inviting pressure onto your shoulders.

The big day will arrive and you will realize that a whole host of friends and relatives are party to your quitting smoking, keeping tabs on your progress and looking over your shoulder. You could inadvertently spin a web of expectation. My concern for you would be that now, with so many people in on your journey, you will be trying to keep others happy, too. Remember what I said earlier about quitting for yourself? Quitting smoking is your thing, your aim, your goal. Whilst telling the world might help bolster your confidence, it might also mean you end up trying to quit for others. And that, as I have said, is a big no-no. This is a selfish thing. It must be for you. Noble as it is to quit for someone else, at some point you will smoke because the quitting becomes about other things. I know. I remember quitting for my wife after she fell pregnant. After a while I fell back into smoking, hiding the truth from her. Even a baby on the way wasn't enough to keep me from the tobacco. By quitting solely for my wife I was an addict simply holding out.

Start to build up a loathing of smoking (you should already hate it, anyway). Believe me, its not hard. Holding on to any notion of pleasure will make quitting needlessly tough. See smoking as it is – a filthy chemical addiction that is destroying your health and fitness. I sincerely hope and expect you to already feel like this about cigarettes, but even so, really start to gear your mind towards quitting. In the past I have virtually blocked the idea of quitting out of my mind until the big day arrived and, as a result, felt underprepared. This time put everything into it. You will reap what you sow.

Use this time to think hard about everything I have said. But don't just take me at my word. Start really looking at these images of supposed Hollywood glamour involving smoking and seeing them as they are: an advert for life-long addiction. Start looking at smokers carefully and you will soon see that they are not enjoying themselves; they are simply self-administering a drug necessary for their peace of mind. Non-smokers don't have to do it. They don't have to stand in the freezing cold or driving rain or knee-deep snow, puffing away on a blend of chemicals. See these smokers as drug addicts forced to smoke and accept you are one of them. But not for much longer.

17. Quitting Smoking

'Nicotine patches are great. Stick one over each eye and you can't find your cigarettes.'

~Anonymous

DON'T WORRY. I'M NOT going to ask you to quit smoking now. In fact, I'm not going to ask you to quit smoking at all. That's your call. This advice is simply for when you are ready. Besides, I'm not finished quite yet. I hope, however, you are feeling confident about breaking away from your addiction and never going back. You are on the precipice of a new life, a life of health and well-being, untainted by the noxious chemical realities of smoking.

In this chapter I want to talk you through that big day when you say goodbye to smoking and those few tentative days that follow. It is a strange time. You have probably been there many times before, going half mad because you want to smoke yet desperately holding out. Don't worry. As long as you understand your addiction and have decided you simply can't smoke anymore, you will be fine. Just keep the right perception.

So, after all the talking, the planning, the dreaming, the day has arrived. You are finally ready to throw away your cigarettes and join the ranks of the non-smoker. This is a time of positivity and hope and excitement. You are breaking away from a filthy, dangerous addiction for good. This is what you want. Quitting smoking will be a dream fulfilled. Forget all those failures that have gone before. This time is for keeps. You will never go back as long as, from the very start, you keep the right attitude.

Ensuring you get off to the best start is very important. As I said earlier, timing is critical. You will, I trust, have identified a quiet and stress-free period of your life, a time when your days are running at a constant. Remember, by choosing this time you are making life far easier on yourself. There can not be anything to distract you from your goal. Now you have identified a good period of your life to quit, you must choose the right time of day. Yes, that's right. This is a small point but it will set you off in good stead. It worked for me.

Smoke your last cigarette around late afternoon: tea-time or thereabouts. This is what I did and I found it a very useful tactic. Spend the morning and early afternoon thinking hard about everything I have told you. Re-read my words if you so wish. Make this a day of reflection, a day of deep sole-searching. You are on the edge of fulfilling your dream – make sure you completely understand where you are. Ensure you have that all-important correct attitude. Have absolutely no doubt about what you're doing. The fact smoking is a waste of time, a chemical addiction that has been fooling you and destroying you for years, should be crystal clear in your mind. Feel this truth, breathe it, understand it. Let it settle in.

Another advantage to quitting at this time of day is that the following morning you will already be in the mind-set of a non-smoker. You won't be starting from scratch. This can prove, as it did for me, a huge psychological boost. Start that first full day of non-smoking with a positive sense of purpose. You are now in the process of freeing yourself of the addiction you loathe.

Smoke every cigarette that last day as consciously as

possible. Taste – really *taste* – the acrid fumes. Consider that the cigarette companies have loaded the cigarette with additives, such as sugar, to make it more bearable and it is still eye-wateringly disgusting. Realize there is no benefit whatsoever to what you are doing. Realize you are sucking in these horrible noxious fumes needlessly. Glory in the fact that this forced activity, this addiction you so hate, is about to end. Forever.

Perhaps in the past you have smoked that 'last' cigarette with something close to dread, or perhaps a degree of fond sentimentality. You have been conditioned to see the cigarette as a trusty friend and that now you are parting company life will never be quite the same. But now, when the time comes to smoke that last cigarette, smoke it with the disgust and contempt it deserves and toss it away with glee. Good riddance!

Bear in mind that cravings will surface. As long as you retain the right perspective, however, these moments will not bother you. I remember only too well that fleeting feeling of 'I want a cigarette', that brief yet strong urge. But keep in mind that cravings are purely emotional. You are in charge, not them. See them for what they are and they will vanish as quickly as they arrived. Don't fear cravings; understand them, expect them, discard them. Every time you swat a craving aside you recondition your mind further towards that of a non-smoker. Just keep the right attitude and perspective

Most of you, I daresay, will encounter other smokers. In a world where well over a billion people smoke, they are virtually unavoidable. Whatever you do, don't start to look upon these smokers with envy. There is nothing – *absolutely nothing* – to feel jealous about. Don't just see that single cigarette they are smoking at that moment. See the thousands of fags they will have to smoke, whether they want to or not. Do they seem happy to be puffing away? Probably not. Their throat will doubtless already be raw from the previous cigarettes. You remember that feeling, don't you? You remember that saturation point where you felt your whole body was riddled with smoke? You will be free from it soon. That smoker you see isn't. You've escaped the prison but that smoker, unfortunately, remains in the trap.

During the early days, you will probably reach for your cigarettes, only to remember you have quit and that there is an empty space once occupied by that familiar packet with the lighter atop. In the past these moments would likely have sparked a strong craving – they did for me. Perhaps it was a moment like this – where you felt down and deprived – that made you cave in and smoke last time. Your brain, don't forget, has been programmed to expect its fix, its rush of dopamine, an end to the itchiness. When it doesn't get its due, it will complain. But this is natural. You are in the process of resetting that automatic reaction, but it won't happen overnight. Stay strong and believe in what you are doing. This is a fantastic, life-changing time. You are sowing the seeds of future health and happiness. Just keep in mind the truth about nicotine. It is a con trick and it won't work on you any more.

Before you arrive at your quitting date, you need to be thoroughly prepared. This is too important, too crucial to your future health, to leave anything to chance. I have summarized everything you need to know before you quit for good:

1) Make sure you understand fully the physical side of

your addiction. Remember that when you take a drag on that cigarette the alkaloid nicotine (which, don't forget, is a neurotoxin designed to protect the tobacco plant from hungry insects) is stealthily transported to your brain and, once there, plays havoc with your neurological processes by mimicking the neurotransmitter acetylcholine. Another neurotransmitter, dopamine, is in turn released in robust quantities, giving you a heightened feeling of satisfaction and a sense of reward, similar to when we eat food or make love. But it is a falsehood, a chemical lie. Tobacco smoke is not satisfactory or rewarding. It is noxious and disgusting.

Also remember that a cigarette reduces the withdrawal symptoms brought about by both your previous cigarette and the weight of psychological conditioning you have received since birth. The cigarette gives you a little respite before returning you to that familiar state of itchiness and agitation. Can you think of anything more pointless?

2) You must be seeing tobacco addiction as it really is. You must remove the smokescreen. Open your eyes and really look. Think hard. You are addicted to the leaves of the tobacco plant, which, once dried and cured and finely chopped – and set in a paper tube – you set fire to and breathe in the resultant fumes. These fumes contain, among other poisons, arsenic, cadmium, carbon monoxide and, most crucially, a highly toxic alkaloid called nicotine that in high doses will kill but in smaller doses creates psychoactive effects in the brain that lead to a life of addiction. That is the bottom line. Nice, eh?

3) Bear in mind that through years of lighting up you have conditioned your brain to expect nicotine at certain

times throughout the day. With tea, coffee, alcohol; during breaks at work; after long car journeys; before making a telephone call. You have spun this complex web of associations, each one triggering a strong desire to smoke. But with effort and focus these triggers can be reversed. You can smash these associations and free your mind but it will not happen overnight. The correct mind-set is essential.

4) You will get cravings, but it is our attitude towards them that keep us imprisoned in our addiction. See these cravings for what they really are: moments where a seemingly fond memory of smoking makes you feel a little uptight and itchy, which your brain interprets as *I want a cigarette*. The more you are able to see smoking in its true light the less these cravings will occur and the less they will bother you when they do. These brief urges to smoke are part of the process of healing body and mind. Stay positive.

5) Make sure you have picked a quiet, 'normal' time in your life to quit smoking. By doing this you are stacking the chips in your favour. The smoking triggers you receive will be familiar – you get the same cravings at these same moments every day. Only this time you will let the urges pass instead of breathing in poisonous smoke to make them go away.

Trying to quit smoking during a time of stress and uncertainty is a recipe for relapse. Your mind needs to be fully on the job, so to speak. Quitting smoking should be your biggest priority. You could be saving your very life – it doesn't get more important than that. If you can't lend your full attention to quitting then put it off till you can.

The last thing you need is a false start.

6) Quit because you can see the naked truth about smoking and have no desire to smoke anymore. The idea that you are being tricked by the chemical properties within tobacco should spur you on to a life of freedom. Quitting smoking solely to save money or repair your health is sensible and very noble but sadly misguided. You already know the health risks – you know people die from smoking – but you are still puffing away. Cigarettes could treble in value within a day and you would still smoke. Only the truth about tobacco – that it offers nothing more than a brief chemical impression of satisfaction and that you simply don't need it – will open those gates and set you free.

7) Prepare thoroughly for quitting smoking. Make sure you have left nothing to chance. You don't want to have to quit again. Get rid of all smoking paraphernalia from your home; you don't need those ashtrays and lighters any more. Ensure the truth about smoking is crystal clear in your head. Is the time right? Are you 100% confident? Prepare well and nothing can stop you achieving a life free from tobacco. This time it is for keeps.

8) And finally, remember that quitting smoking is the single greatest gift you can bestow upon yourself. You are handing yourself health, fitness and well-being and, most of all, the chance to ditch the pointless addiction that is dragging you down further every day. You are taking back your life. As long as you continue to see smoking in its ugly true light, you will never regret your decision.

The time will fairly fly by. The days will quickly melt into weeks. Smoking will seem more and more alien as time advances. As your breathing and general health slowly improve you will begin to see just how far down tobacco has dragged you. There is no nicer feeling than realizing that you no longer need or desire cigarettes.

But we are getting ahead of ourselves. You have probably been here before. The trouble is, at some point, you have returned to smoking. This time that cannot happen. *Don't* let it happen.

Let us see how we need never go back.

18. Never Going Back

'Stopping smoking is for life – not just for the New Year.'

~Anonymous

SO WHAT NOW? You have finally stopped smoking. Your breathing is beginning to improve, as are your energy levels. There isn't that stench of stale smoke clinging to your clothes to feel conscious about. You have a little extra money in your pocket. But still ... there's just something missing, a feeling of emptiness. Maybe, seeing as you have done so well, you could treat yourself to one fag, just the one – even if it is to prove you are no longer addicted. One can't hurt, can it?

The key to avoiding a return to smoking is to ensure you don't end up thinking about smoking in a positive light. This chapter is perhaps the most crucial section of the book. Quitting smoking is one thing; staying there is quite another. I daresay most of us have, at some point, tried to quit smoking. If you're reading this book then you probably weren't successful. Don't worry, that will change. But now we must look at why ex-smokers go back to the cigarettes after long periods of abstention and make sure we don't follow suit.

I found this idea that smokers could return to smoking after years of freedom one of the biggest obstacles when quitting. How was I ever going to be happy again? How could I ever be free? These were questions that dogged my previous attempts to quit smoking. I couldn't see a way forward. I thank the heavens I did find a way through in the end. You will too. I can see now that these smokers who return to smoking after years of abstention have spent those years clinging to the notion that smoking is something necessary and pleasurable. They have exhibited tremendous willpower in fighting those urges and, over time, their addicted minds have come to accept the absence of tobacco. But not completely.

Hiding in the undergrowth, a stubborn splinter of their addiction has lain in wait. At some point they have fantasized about smoking, generating a craving. That craving has led to others. Over time their desire to light up has snowballed and eventually, during a weak moment, they have smoked. No doubt they kicked themselves once the smoke hit their throat and the nicotine flooded their brain, but by then it was too late. You see, nicotine addicts can't smoke. Ever. Just one cigarette will see you sliding back into the cycle of smoking despair.

Armed with the knowledge that smoking is nothing but a pointless chemical addiction, you will quit smoking in a position of authority and remain there. You will understand your addiction and be ready to put down any rogue thoughts of smoking. As time goes on, this resolve will strengthen. Unlike those smokers who turned to smoking after years of abstention, you will never need to, safe in the knowledge that tobacco never did anything for you, and never possibly could.

The guidelines below – provided you follow them closely – will see you stay smoke-free:

1) Never, ever touch another cigarette. This might sound somewhat obvious but you would be surprised at the amount of smokers who quit for a while only to then think they are safe to smoke. No ex-addict is safe to begin using again. If you smoke you will quickly return to your old

levels of consumption. Those reward pathways and associations will spring into life and hook you in. All your effort and planning will be for nothing. You are quitting smoking because you no longer wish to smoke. In which case, don't go back. Ever.

2) Keep the right attitude, always. See smoking for what it is: a filthy, deadly addiction that has robbed you of years of health and fitness and well-being. You never smoked for pleasure. You smoked because you were addicted to nicotine and had no choice but to light up filthy fag after filthy fag, puffing away desperately through colds and chest infections. Keep your thoughts focused. Wake up each morning and consider how fortunate you are to be removed from smoking. Keep that crucial perception intact and you will never feel the need to smoke.

3) If you find yourself overeating, do not use this as a justification to smoke. Puffing away on noxious gases isn't a good diet aid. Try to eat as healthily as possible if you're consuming a lot. Also, a little gentle exercise will not only help burn away those extra calories but will release endorphins, helping you to feel better about things. Putting on weight is never ideal. But is a life of chemical addiction, a life of dependency to nicotine a worthwhile alternative? Of course not. Don't panic about your weight. Eat as sensibly as you can and enjoy life without tobacco.

4) Get out there and live life. Our existence on this planet is a one-off, our brief chance in the story of humanity to love and laugh and marvel at the beauty that surrounds us. Life is not perfect, but it has many moments of perfection. Enjoy these times without having to breathe

in the poisonous fumes from cigarettes. Use your fleeting time on earth wisely and fully and never blight your existence by being a drug addict. You are free now. Stay that way.

5) Remember, other smokers will seriously envy you, even if they pretend they don't. No one really wants to be trapped in a cycle of addiction. Most smokers want to be rid of cigarettes but are too scared of what life will be like without their longtime companion. They hate their addiction just as you hated yours. If they want to quit, share with them my advice. But don't preach. There is nothing more irritating than an ex-smoker who, after being without tobacco for a matter of days, starts wagging their finger like a stern schoolmaster at smokers – who get enough stick already. Best just to recommend my book and leave it at that.

6) When you get a craving – and you will – go through the breathing routine and question that craving in-depth: how does it really feel? Is it hurting? Do I want to smoke now I know the truth? Remember: a craving is just the old programming kicking in. Your brain needs time to accept the positive changes you are making. Your poor mind was tricked, don't forget, into seeing tobacco as precious. Keep the truth in mind and your subconscious mind will follow suit. See these urges and desires as part of the recuperation process. Don't fear them – they last minutes and can't hurt you. As time goes on, cravings will virtually go for good. Each craving defied is a big stride towards freedom.

Going back to smoking will be a grave mistake, quite literally. Anyone returning to smoking after years will tell you how gutted they are to be trapped once again. They must now go through the quitting process right from scratch. If only they could have had the foresight to avoid this state of affairs.

Don't be one of these people. You know exactly why you smoked, and this knowledge will keep you safe. Even now I have the occasional thought of smoking. But I am philosophical. If I smoked now I know it would taste awful and bring on a coughing fit. My brain would flood with nicotine and I would reawaken those dormant reward pathways. I would cause myself anguish and stress at the thought of having to quit all over again. That cigarette would just be pointless now – it always was.

Consider this. If you are tempted at any time to light up think first of the options you have. Your first option is not to smoke, by a country mile the most desirable option. By saying no you are reinforcing your new smoke-free life and retaining the correct mind-set. You are keeping on the road to freedom, a road you were desperate to set out on. Option two is to smoke and then give up again. Why bother? You already are a non-smoker. Why smoke then quit again? How pointless. You can't keep doing that, can you? Do you want to spend the rest of your life constantly having to fall victim to smoking, over and again? Option three is to smoke and not quit. In other words, be forced to smoke till the day you die. Do you want that? Of course you don't. The mere thought is horrendous. But that is what will happen if you don't quit and stay that way. There are no other options.

Whenever you think about smoking, treat that thought as a positive reminder of how you changed your life for the better. You were an addict trapped in a cycle of misery but now you are free.

And you will never go back.

19. End Game

'It's easy to quit smoking. I've done it hundreds of times.'

~Mark Twain

THIS BOOK HAS BEEN ABOUT something that in principle is very simple. When you think about it, all you need to do is never smoke another cigarette. It is not like some unseen force will physically pluck a cigarette from a box, stuff it in your mouth and light it. The only way you will smoke is if you want to. If you let the lies of tobacco begin to encroach on the truth, then you will become a prime candidate for relapse. I don't want this to happen to you.

In the previous chapter, I went through all the things you need to know and keep fresh in your mind if you are to avoid a miserable reunion with tobacco. But the passage of time can chip away at our best intentions. Years from now, when smoking hasn't entered your mind in a long time, you could well find yourself suddenly standing on the edge of relapse. If you can keep alive and vivid in your mind the reality of smoking – that it is a chemical lie and that there is nothing inherently pleasurable about it – then I doubt you will ever smoke again. But what if your resolve slips?

Remember, the point is to remain a non-smoker, not just to quit and eventually relapse. The rot can sometimes take weeks to set in. You start with a faint thought of smoking, a brief image of pleasure. You swat it aside but it keeps coming back, stronger and stronger. The faint tracks of addiction left in your subconscious mind begin to re-emerge. Slowly you begin to rationalize smoking, using spurious logic as to why lighting up isn't such a bad idea.

The deleterious effects of your addiction are now history. Your breathing in normal, your fingers unstained, your teeth white. The raw smokiness of tobacco in your throat is too vague to recall. With inexorable force the reality of smoking edges nearer and nearer.

I have been here before. You might recall me telling you how I quit for six months, only to return to smoking. There was a slow undoing of all the logic I had employed, all the fortifications I had thrown up. I finally lit that cigarette. The noxious smoke hit the back of my throat and brought about a prolonged coughing fit. I remember thinking how vile it tasted. Next, I went extremely lightheaded as the nicotine flooded my brain. Already I was regretting what I had done. I asked myself why I had done it. What was the point? There was no stress to relieve, and even if there had been the cigarette could not have helped. I didn't need a boost in any way. I smoked because I thought it would end the growing mental torture of not smoking. But it did nothing.

The sense of regret I felt was all-consuming. I had gone six whole months without touching a cigarette and suddenly, for reasons lost to me, I was back into tobacco's fold. I was furious with myself. Over the next few days I reawakened my addiction. Smoking was extremely unpleasant at first, every drag raw on my throat and chest. This shows the pure pointlessness of smoking: I actually had to work hard to reacquaint myself with the cigarette, puffing away against my better judgment to get that false chemical fix. Soon enough I was back to twenty-a-day and hating it. Once again my chest was painful in the morning. My mouth was constantly scummy. My clothes and hair and hands bore the constant stench of stale smoke, a smell that, as a non-smoker, I had come to detest. Smoking was back with a vengeance.

This is how it happens. You think you are free and tobacco plays a killer move in the end game and brings you crashing down. That being the case, are all of us destined to be hooked back into the addiction, whether we want to or not? The answer is emphatically *no*.

Just think about it. If you return to smoking you will sooner or later try to escape again. The second I went back to smoking I was thinking ahead to my next bid for freedom. Do you really want to live a life in which you are continually falling in and out of addiction? Of course not. You want to be free and stay that way. Bear in mind that if you smoke you will wish you were still a non-smoker. You know you will. Don't see that single cigarette. It will not help you. It will lead you back into the addiction you worked hard to escape from. If you truly want to be a non-smoker then at some point *you will have to quit smoking and never go back.*

You can't keep putting it off. I have said in this book that I will not pressure you into quitting smoking, and I stand by that. But if you really desire an end to this nightmare, in which you want to smoke yet want to quit, you must get real. The only way to do it is *to do it.* Imagine lying on your death bed regretting never being able to quit. Think of how you would resent smoking for enslaving you for life. But it doesn't have to be that way.

I'm not saying I will look back at my life and see no regrets. There will be things I wish I had not done. But I know now that when my time is up I will look back and give thanks that I was able to purge the curse of smoking from my life. We get one life, nothing more. Don't waste it by going back to smoking. You know deep down you can't continue to smoke. In which case, stop doing it.

Society is moving away from smoking. One day it will be gone for good. Don't stay hooked to these foul things for the rest of your life. Take back control. Remember everything you now know about smoking and use it to stay smoke-free.

Live, love, laugh and, most of all, be free.

AUTHOR'S NOTE

I want to take this opportunity to thank every smoker I have ever spoken to. You have helped me build up a picture of smoking. That picture turned into *Quit Smoking & Never Go Back*. Any factual errors are purely my own. I'd like also to thank my long-suffering wife Laura for putting up with me during the tortuous process of writing this book. I can't promise I won't do it again.

I hope all of you can remain smoke-free and happy for life. If you would like to share any thoughts with me then I would love to hear from you. You can contact me at paulecclesx@msn.com.

Remember, don't be fooled by tobacco. Re-read this book as many times as you might need to and keep in mind the core message: smoking is simply the process of inhaling fumes from burning tobacco leaves, which contain a chemical called nicotine that causes acute addiction – for life, if you don't do something about it.

Don't be an addict. Be free.

AUTHOR BIOGRAPHY

Paul Eccles was born in Birmingham, UK, in 1981. He did a variety of job roles after leaving school, including stints as a barman, building site labourer and shop assistant before settling in the care profession. Paul always had an interest in writing, and when he quit smoking he found an outlet for his passion that evolved into his first book, *Quit Smoking & Never Go Back*. He lives in Cornwall with his wife and four children.

www.ingramcontent.com/pod-product-compliance
Lightning Source LLC
Chambersburg PA
CBHW020257290526
45784CB00003B/1282